the Conscious Pregnancy

A SPIRITUAL & PRACTICAL APPROACH TO CREATING A ZEN BABY

PRAISE

"Shivani's book left me at the edge of my seat. It was exciting, enticing, interesting, and full of valuable information. Now when I am ready to have a baby, I will feel prepared and at ease. I look forward to trying many things Shivani mentioned. I highly recommend you read this, whether you are a first-time mom or a sixth-time mom, it will still help you!"

ASHLEY AGELOFF, *Thermographic Technician and*

Nutritional Coach at YourLimitlessHealth.com

"It feels like I read this book in just one breath! With her knowledge, passion, and insight, Shivani brings sacredness and empowerment back to new mamas. Pregnancy is properly realized as a spiritual journey, and *The Conscious Pregnancy* provides everything we need for this sacred process."

WANDA KRUSZYNSKA, *Ayurvedic Massage Therapist*

"*The Conscious Pregnancy* takes the reader on a journey of the East meets the West. Through the personal experience of pain and triumph, it provides guidelines, principles, and practical tools for the wellness of both mother and baby on every level: Body, Mind, and Spirit. Through timeless wisdom, we learn how to intuitively embrace the oldest known form of medicine in the world and are lovingly taught that it is possible for any mother to create a Zen baby of her own."

KAMILLE DAWN TIRZAH, *Health, Fitness and*

Nutrition Specialist and Creator of Lean Body Principles

"Shivani is clearly passionate about ensuring women have a peaceful and positive pregnancy that leads to the healthiest of outcomes for both mother and child. Pregnancy is often fraught with questions and anxiety, and she has drawn from her own experiences to offer practical tips to navigate that journey."

GAURI AGARWAL, *M.D., F.A.C.P., Associate Regional Dean of*

Medical Curriculum, University of Miami - Miller School of Medicine

"*The Conscious Pregnancy* is the book women—who are having fertility problems or are interested in learning about the modern medicine approach to pregnancy—have been waiting for. Reading Shivani's own story of hardship and growth experiences showcases the difficult side of pregnancy and how, with small lifestyle changes and awareness, we can learn to have healthy pregnancies for our own bodies and not just healthy babies in today's toxic world. A must read for any woman interested in becoming pregnant in today's stressful environment."

NEHA GUPTA, *Author of The Four Year Plan,*

Creator of College Shortcuts and CEO of Elite Private Tutors

"This is the book of the moment for pregnant women and couples, midwives, doulas, and educators. *The Conscious Pregnancy* is an empowering book offering a spiritual and practical approach for the modern-day woman. In it, there is a lot of helpful advice, positive discussion, and support about having a blissful pregnancy."

DEVINA VADERA-BHANDARI, *Founder, My Little Pudding*

"*The Conscious Pregnancy* is very eye-opening and a must-read for any women considering having a child—and for almost anyone in general. I did NOT grow up in a green home, nor around anyone that was conscientious about everything that is brought to light in this book. As a two-time cancer survivor, now getting ready to have a hysterectomy in a few weeks for endometrial cancer, I wish I had this insight when I was younger. I have already changed many things in my life as a result of what I went through over the past five years, but will undoubtedly utilize this powerful book and the messages in it to make even more changes for the well-being of my daughter."

SHERYL LAU, *Personal Trainer & Certified Spin/Kickboxing/Mat Pilates Instructor, Former National Level Figure Competitor, Operations Manager and Corporate Wellness Director*

"*The Conscious Pregnancy* is a beautiful book for any woman who is either looking to be pregnant or just cares about herself. The title is Conscious Pregnancy, but the information inside is for any woman who is interested in living a healthier life through truly simple habits and choices. Shivani shares her vulnerable experiences through pregnancies and birth while giving suggestions that make you see you have options that will be better for the baby and give your life more peace and joy in the process. Instead of overwhelming the reader with all the things that can go wrong or every nuance of pregnancy you can experience — that's been done before — it provides a great attitude and mindset for living a happy life, pregnant or not."

AMY LYN D'ALESIO, *President, Creative Types*

"I'm super excited about the release of this book and cannot wait to give it as a gift to my girlfriends who are currently or trying to become pregnant. I definitely wish I could have had a resource like this, especially during my second pregnancy, when I seriously struggled with finding a balance between taking care of my first son, not falling behind on my work, and taking care of myself. I literally worked with contractions until 6:00 PM on the day my son was born because I *had* to finish my work before going on maternity leave. During my leave, I even rushed back to work without taking the necessary time for my baby and me to bond — something that I believe still affects our relationship three years later, and I fear will have a lifetime effect. I wish I'd had someone I trusted telling me to slow down, live in the moment, and take care of myself and my son without feeling guilty. I thank Shivani for making it a priority for moms to have a navigation tool during life's most beautiful journey — becoming a mother."

ADRIANA GONZALEZ, *Attorney, Mom of two boys, President of Palm Beach County Hispanic Bar Association, Active community member*

"While being pregnant is thrilling, the responsibility of a growing baby can provoke anxiety on many different levels. When had I learned I was pregnant with my first child, I was excited and also very nervous. My anxiety levels manifested into various ailments I'd later experience throughout my pregnancy and delivery. If this book was around back then, I think it would have definitely assuaged my concerns. It is wonderful to know we are in charge of our health and we do not need to be pressured into using the conventional practices of modern medicine. I took the epidural both times and am still dealing with the repercussions of my choices even now, 13 years later. This book has been an eye-opener for me—very empowering. It will definitely encourage anyone trying to conceive to have a look within themselves, listen to their bodies, be conscious and present in the journey, and find the wonderful natural methods they can use. I can't wait to buy a handful of copies of this book to gift all my friends who are pregnant right now or trying to get pregnant!"

SNEHA RODRIGUEZ, *Mother to two boys in Boynton Beach, FL*

"Shivani is a passionate visionary and teacher with an old soul. Her work is a reflection of what she wants for her family, friends, and loved ones. She has inspired me to live life better in all ways. Every time I talk to her or read her work, I learn something new. She is a gift."

LAUREN-MAY MALIS, *Publisher, Palm Beach Woman Magazine, CEO, Luxe*

Partners II, Author of I fell off my Pradas (Fall 2016)

the Conscious Pregnancy

A SPIRITUAL & PRACTICAL APPROACH TO CREATING A ZEN BABY

SHIVANI GUPTA

The Conscious Pregnancy:
A Spiritual and Practical Approach
to Creating a Zen Baby

Contact information at www.ShivaniGupta.com

Cover and Interior Design: David B. Lee
Author Photograph: Bea Byers
Editor: Berni Xiong

ISBN: 978-0-9974062-9-0

To my husband, my two magical children, and family,
Your love and support made this book
possible and me a better person.

FOREWORD

I wish I'd had this book when I was pregnant. I was 28 when I became unexpectedly pregnant with my son Daniel and I was completely unable to prepare ahead. It was quite a shock as I hadn't planned on getting pregnant and wasn't sure that I could even get pregnant. Also, this pregnancy came at a particularly stressful time in my own life. I was working full time and driving hundreds of miles every weekend to complete my acupuncture clinical training.

Oh, how I wish I had had Shivani's book to encourage me to treat this pregnancy with the reverence it deserved. And to treat myself with the kindness and compassion I needed. And to follow my instincts. I am sure that my son's birth would have been an easier experience, but more importantly, I am certain that my little baby would have had a calmer and happier start to his life.

I wrote the book (*Homeopathy for Pregnancy, Birth & Your Baby's First Years*) I wish I'd had when I was pregnant. It is full of good healing and homeopathic advice. But I wish I had had *The Conscious Pregnancy* as a companion guide—to help me connect with the spirit of the venture and to deeply question the wisdom of choosing so many stressors at a time when it would have been wiser to back off.

Apart from the aforementioned stressors, I was awash in anxiety and fears, especially about the birth. I couldn't find information or support for my concerns. I was repeatedly told that my worries and fears were unfounded by friends, loved ones, doctors, and acupuncturists. I felt unheard and disempowered.

Every pregnant, birthing or newly-delivered woman will have the experience of being disempowered at some point—whether it's from losing control over important decisions or from being labeled as a difficult patient when expressing fundamental beliefs that vary from their medical professionals. Shivani urges us to stamp our feet and take back our power—to seek medical professionals and hospitals who will listen to us and support our decisions and practices.

Every pregnant woman deserves information in the face of confusion, fear or worry. Kindness in the face of difficulties. Compassion in the face of loss. And, respect in the face of differences of opinion.

I am in love with Shivani and her intrepid heart—especially when it comes to the fierce sheltering she insists on for the little beings that we grow in our "baby palaces." Her depiction of her own culture's rituals and traditions around pregnancy and birth are touching to read—a far cry from the hands-off approach of many Western cultures that leave mothers and babies isolated and fending for themselves.

Shivani touches on many of the hard issues and challenges faced by women and their partners at each and every step of the pregnancy process. She gives clear and straightforward suggestions for dealing with them. I particularly loved the Ayurvedic way with newly-delivered mothers who are encouraged to nurture the baby as if she or he were still inside the womb. This concept opened up a world of possibilities for me—one of many I got from reading this book.

This little book has a huge heart bursting with wise nuggets of gold. It is your insightful mother, your sagacious grandmother, and your intuitive inner voice all rolled into one. All gentleness with a heartfelt firmness of intention.

MIRANDA CASTRO, *FSHom(UK), CCH, RSHom; Best-selling author of Homeopathy for Pregnancy, Birth and Your Baby's First Years; Gainesville, Florida; MirandaCastro.com*

I FELT LIKE A GHOST WALKING

The most common way people give up their power is by thinking they don't have any. - Alice Walker

I gazed at the blip on the screen, saw the expression on the nurse's face, and looked back at the screen. It was incomprehensible. I could not believe my eyes.

"What? Are you telling me there was a baby and now *no* baby?"

She nodded, confirming my fears.

Before this moment, I had learned of a statistic that 40 percent of pregnancies end in miscarriage.

Was this seriously happening to me?

Where did I go wrong?

Was it the wine I had in Italy before I knew I was pregnant?

Over and over, I kept replaying these tapes in my head of how I should have done this or could have done that. I felt shattered and in disbelief, but harping on the past was not going to bring the baby back to me.

"How could I lose the baby? *How?*" I wailed in a voicemail message I left for my sister, Neha, who lived across the country from me. Within hours of leaving that message, Neha was on the next flight to come take care of me. I was going to need all the help I could get to pick up the pieces of my broken spirit.

The Frightful Morning

Before I had learned of my miscarriage, I started spotting that very morning. My husband sensed my trepidation and urged me to visit the doctor, as a precautionary measure. I called Kavita, my sister-in-law and best friend, to ask her to accompany me to the clinic since my husband had to work.

After a grueling two hours in the waiting room, the technician brought me into the exam room and started the abdominal ultrasound. Kavita stayed with me throughout the entire exam, comforting me with soothing words and firmly holding my hand as we kept our eyes peeled on the heartbeat monitor.

"It doesn't look promising. I'll need to have the doctor double-check," the technician hesitantly disclosed.

Kavita took me to lunch to get my mind off of things as we waited for the doctor's final word on the results. Feeling both anxious and restless, I barely ate my soup. We returned to the clinic and waited for another hour before the doctor was ready to see me. Since my obstetrician was out of town, I met with her stand-in. She confirmed the technician's hunch: there was no heartbeat.

Upon hearing the news, my mind went into a haze. I felt emotionally gutted—ripped open with my heart torn out of my chest—and at my wit's end as to how I'd piece myself back together after this.

I recall little of that conversation except for what the doctor instructed me upon leaving the exam: "Your next step is to schedule an appointment with the surgery center to have the fetus removed."

The Dreadful Day

The day continued its downward spiral. After learning I had miscarried the baby, I got shuffled off to a business office to schedule the dilation and curettage (D&C) procedure.

The scheduling manager—who made little effort to console me or show compassion—located the next available appointment time. They could schedule me for the procedure in two days.

Two days?

They want me to wait again?

Is this a joke?

I am a human being, damn it!

I screamed on the inside to no avail.

Delirious from my ghastly morning and infuriated with this cold and uncaring clinical system (which put my last DMV experience to shame!), I was done. No one deserves being treated like a number—especially not after losing a baby.

Then it hit me like a jolt of lightening—my moment of reckoning.

You do not have to do this, Shivani.

Take back your power, now.

I conjured up every last ounce of strength I had left in me after a day in hell and back and gave myself another option.

"Let me get back to you when I make *my* decision," I declared before hightailing out of that dingy office. The scheduling manager carried on to the next person in line—just another day, another surgery (at least that's how it appeared to me). I felt liberated and defeated at the same time.

I immediately called Lorie, my doula (my childbirth coach and supporter), and gave her the news. She responded with exactly what I needed at that moment—kindness and understanding. I also asked her to help me find a new obstetrician. Lorie immediately recommended someone she had worked with at the birthing center. Even though their office closed for the business day, I adamantly wanted to contact my new doctor as soon as possible.

At 5:00 PM, I submitted a message through their website contact form sharing my horrific experience from earlier in the day. Within thirty minutes, the obstetrician's nurse returned my message with a phone call.

"I am so sorry for what is happening to you. This is an urgent matter so Dr. L will see you first thing in the morning."

I am not a proponent of invasive Western medical procedures or drugs unless a situation warrants it. My doula and new obstetrician both seemed to honor my stance on this so I felt comforted that the day would, at least, end with a glimmer of hope—an opportunity to get a second opinion.

The Next Mourning

I wore a black dress to my appointment with Dr. L the next morning. I was in mourning. Void of emotion. Invisible. I felt like a ghost walking into a room full of people who couldn't see me.

Neha, who had flown in the night before, was my rock for day two. From the moment we left my house through to the very end of my appointment, everything was a blur for me. As each minute ticked by, I would get lost in a fog. One moment I felt confused and the next moment scared. I became paralyzed by the thoughts racing through my mind as we anticipated Dr. L's findings:

Why is this happening to me?

Will I ever be able to have kids again?

This was not part of the plan.

I was excited and ready to have my baby.

What did I do wrong?

I hope this does not hurt.

Dr. L completed the ultrasound and confirmed there was no heartbeat. He said so with kind eyes and compassion. He advised me that I had two options, but a surgical procedure to remove the fetus would be unnecessary. I emailed the news to my in-laws before I left the clinic. By the time I had arrived home, half of them were already at my house to greet and console me. They illuminated my day despite the devastating circumstances that had unfolded the last 24 hours.

We often underestimate how much our family means to us until we're faced with debilitating times like these. Though I felt so alone and as if I had crumbled into a thousand pieces, I also felt empowered because of the love and support my family gave me when I needed it most.

The Silver Lining

That night, Neha and I lay in bed together. We relaxed, watched TV together, and then I passed it—the *almost* baby. We hear stories about others having miscarriages, but we never think it can happen to us. It's hard to explain the experience, other than this sensation of immediately feeling better. I was sad to be among the 40 percent, but I believe tragedy can be a breeding ground for opportunity.

Though I wish this experience on no one, mine taught me to ask better questions of myself and of my health care practitioners. Today, I am an Ayurvedic Practitioner and Healer, and the proud mother of two healthy and inquisitive bundles of joy.

If you're looking for a *how-to* guide on the A to Z of pregnancy, put this book down because you will be disappointed. This book does not have all the answers—no book does.

The Conscious Pregnancy represents so much more than a personal aspiration to tell my story or an attempt to give you advice. There is no way I've got it all figured out as I'm still navigating motherhood, but think of this book as a cautionary tale written by your protective big sister.

I handcrafted this guide for you because it's something I wish I had in my possession long ago, before becoming a mom. Back then, when my body would tell me to slow down, I would kick it into overdrive. When I second-guessed myself, I would defer important health decisions to other people.

I feel the weight of the world sits on my shoulders to advocate for you—the new mom—and for the Zen Baby you'll bring into this world. *The Conscious Pregnancy* is both my message and encouragement to challenge what you think you already know, to question the dogma fed to you, and to make conscious choices based on *your* fundamental beliefs and values.

Introduction:

YOU RUN THE SHOW

We may act sophisticated and worldly but I believe we feel safest when we go inside ourselves and find home, a place where we belong and maybe the only place we really do. - Maya Angelou

The Conscious Pregnancy is a far cry from the ideal that you must have a perfect pregnancy. In this book, I encourage you to throw away perfection and instead make deliberate choices every day to prepare your mind, spirit, and body for a healthy and happy baby and a conscious rest of your life.

What is a Zen Baby?

A Zen Baby is created by a mother who prioritizes the loving energy and healthy intentions to nurture herself and the fetus growing inside her womb. A Zen Baby is equipped for a vigorous life—less prone to chronic illness or disease — because of the conscious choices the mother has made before, during and after pregnancy.

The concept for *The Conscious Pregnancy* framework was born in the same delivery room where I gave birth to Anya, my first child. Despite having a healthy pregnancy, I experienced a traumatizing childbirth. Anya had arrived seven days late and spent ten days in the Neonatal Intensive Care Unit (NICU) with a collapsed lung.

To help you understand why this experience cemented my belief that I could no longer leave my health decisions in someone else's hands, first, let me give you some background.

The Inexhaustible Anya

My husband is a doctor of Western medicine and, naturally, his views are heavily influenced by Western practices. Though I was born and bred in the Western world, I was influenced by Eastern philosophies and experimented with alternative healing practices since I was a little girl. Because of our disparate views, my husband and I were forced to make compromises when we decided to have a baby.

I initially pushed hard for a natural birth. I wanted a midwife to support me during pregnancy and to deliver my baby. Though midwives are recognized as qualified and trained specialists for pregnancy and childbirth, my husband preferred for our baby to be delivered by an obstetrician in a hospital. That one request was his only request.

I conceded on the natural birth idea and determined I would, at least, get a doula—someone who could advocate for me through labor and delivery and help me avoid any unnecessary interventions or a C-section. In return, my husband gave me free reign to make 100 percent of the choices concerning the pregnancy.

When we arrived at the home stretch of my pregnancy, I was still not going into labor. What made matters worse, my whole body erupted into an itchy rash. I scratched my belly to the point of bleeding, which gave me an inkling that my body was no longer tolerating this pregnancy well. Then, I had a realization.

Oh no, I might have to get induced!

I had learned in a HypnoBirthing® class (using hypnotherapy to aid the birthing process) I took during my pregnancy that the baby would decide when she wants to be born. If we interceded, we could perpetuate problems or face possible complications.

I was apprehensive about inducing the labor because I didn't want to play Mother Nature. My husband, on the other hand, feared my health would deteriorate if I waited any longer to give birth to the baby. The battle between the East and West reared its ugly head again. After weighing the pros and cons of each decision, we came to an agreement together: I would get induced.

We arrived at the hospital for the scheduled procedure the very next Thursday at 8:00 in the morning. They administered the epidural — an anesthesia that is injected into the spinal nerves to numb the pain of childbirth—another procedure I was initially against. I had printed my original birth plan for my doula and me to follow, but nothing was going as I had planned. It was a suffocating feeling to lose control over such monumental decisions.

Lorie reassured me, "Whatever happens at birth, let go of your preconceived notions. Let go of control. It may not be going the way you want, but accept and enjoy whatever happens during this process."

By 4:00 PM, it was time to push. I pushed as hard as I could, but it was difficult to feel anything as I was numb from my belly to toes. I have no idea what I would have done without Lorie helping me through this.

Thirty minutes later, I gave birth to my daughter. I held her for only a few seconds. Within minutes, my new beautiful baby girl was being carted off to the NICU. With anguish in his eyes, my husband looked at the team and then gazed back at me.

"No!" he firmly instructed them. "You will give the child to her mother first."

It was such a powerful statement he made. To me, it meant that my husband understood how hard I had worked before and during my pregnancy to prepare for this special day.

Despite our differences, he knew the whole birthing experience was crucial for me—it would shape my first memories as a new mom. He also grasped the severity of the situation as I did. What if we missed out on the opportunity to send loving energies to our daughter before anything else went wrong? He and I both knew we would regret it for the rest of our lives.

As I held my innocent baby girl in my arms, I couldn't help but think I might not ever see her again. I begged everyone to send her love, prayers, and blessings. I asked Neha and my mom to touch her feet. I felt desperate, with no clue what else to do.

Everyone eventually cleared the room and my husband accompanied the baby to the NICU. Unable to move and feeling isolated in my dark lit room, I was devastated that the beautiful baby I had been creating inside me the last nine months was being taken away from me so soon after her arrival.

I remember lying in my bed all alone, spiraling in a sea of somber thoughts. I prayed as hard as I could, begging God, "Please let my baby live." The emotional pain of contemplating the loss of a child was far more unbearable than the physical pain piercing throughout my body after coming off of the epidural.

My husband later returned to the room and escorted me to visit the baby in the NICU. I was horrified by the scene. Here was this tiny baby inside a box and attached to monitors like a lab rat. Her body was covered with tape and needles—tubes protruding from her nostrils.

My heart sank in my chest and my mind took me to dark places.

Is she going to live?

Where's the organic blanket I made for her?

Don't fall in love with her yet, she might not make it.

I stayed in the hospital for two more days just so I could be close to her. I could not bear the thought of leaving my precious newborn at the hospital all by herself. With every waking hour I spent in the hospital, I found myself becoming more aggravated.

My husband and I decided we would finally return home where we could find solace and get some sleep. We returned to the hospital every day to visit the baby in the NICU during the two-hour window in which we were allowed to see her.

I pumped breast milk for her, but they gave her baby formula even when I asked them not to. They kept increasing the amount of formula they fed her though I expressly urged them to stop. I brought the organic soap I had picked out and tested for her, but they did not use that either.

I had relinquished much control during childbirth, so when my requests fell on deaf ears once again, I became exasperated. No mattered how hard I tried, I became so disconnected from the baby I'd been nurturing inside me for over nine months.

Have you ever had a nightmare in which you're shouting for help at the top of your lungs and no one can hear you? That was pretty much the extent of each visit to the NICU. I left the hospital in tears many times—I felt unheard and uninvolved.

This is not an attempt to discount Western practices whatsoever. The hospital staff was following their procedures, and I can understand that. I was very grateful we had an incredible NICU staff that saved her life. What disheartened me about this childbirth experience was getting automatically dismissed because, "pregnant women and new moms are just emotional and hormonal," as I've heard stated before.

Whether or not my perception was accurate, I felt misunderstood and placed in a box: viewed as a defiant mom who aimed to disrupt the medical system each time I expressed my fundamental beliefs. Though I was an authority on organic pregnancy and organic baby products (through my experience running *Sama Baby*, my organic cotton children's clothing line that sold in Whole Foods stores and boutiques across the United States), I felt powerless most days as a new mom in the hospital.

As Lorie taught me when we entered the hospital, I had to focus on what I could control no matter how minor the decision seemed. For me, it was less about being right and more about being heard. When I decided to work within the constraints of the system, I was able to bridge the divide between the West and the East.

Regardless of which direction your views lean, I encourage you (new or existing mom) to ask better questions of yourself and of your healthcare team.

It was a joyous occasion for me when I finally was able to line the baby's box with an organic blanket—I even got to put a *Sama Baby* hat on her head. I also brought in a small iPod and speaker I had purchased for her nursery to play for her my favorite yoga music from my prenatal classes and daily meditations. I decided that if I couldn't stay with the baby, I would do my best to provide a soothing environment for her by muffling the sounds of the beeping machines. Since my husband and I were unable to stay with her 24/7, I placed a picture of us right in her box so she could see us watching over her—to feel close to us even when we were away.

By day ten, we were told our baby's health was in stable condition. We could bring our daughter home and finally give her the name we picked out for her: *Anya*, which means "inexhaustible" and "extraordinary" in Sanskrit.

No mother or newborn baby should go through the ordeal we did. Not all hospitals are created equal. I happened to choose a facility that was misaligned with my views on breastfeeding and organic practices, but I know there are birthing centers that do support these types of values.

I vowed that when I became pregnant again, *I* was going to run the show — all the way to the birthing room. I began developing my own spiritual and practical approach fusing Western practices with ancient Eastern healing modalities. I implemented this framework during my subsequent pregnancy with my son, Aditya, whose pregnancy was night and day compared to Anya's birth. When Aditya was born, everything went without a hitch. Both the pregnancy and childbirth were blissful and beautiful, just as I envisioned they could be.

Five Phases of The Conscious Pregnancy

In this book, I am sharing my framework publicly with the world for the first time. Use these guidelines, not as another rule, but as a compass on your journey towards having a conscious pregnancy and creating a Zen Baby.

The Conscious Pregnancy is comprised of five distinct phases a woman goes through before, during, and after pregnancy:

Building the Baby Palace (Pre-Pregnancy)

The Sad, Sick, and Spent Phase (Trimester One)

The Beautiful, Blessed, and Blissful Phase (Trimester Two)

The Eager, Excruciating, and Equipped Phase (Trimester Three)

The Rebuilding, Restoring, and Renewing Phase (Post-Pregnancy)

As you read the following chapters and apply the tools that make the most sense to you, I urge you to release the guilt we attach to why, what, how, and who we *should* be during pregnancy and childbirth.

This is not an "East versus West" book.

You *can* throw out the rules. You *can* combine the best of both worlds to make decisions that align with your mind, spirit, and body. You, too, *can* have a conscious pregnancy and create a Zen Baby.

You run the show.

CONTENTS

Preparing the Baby Palace

CHAPTER 1:

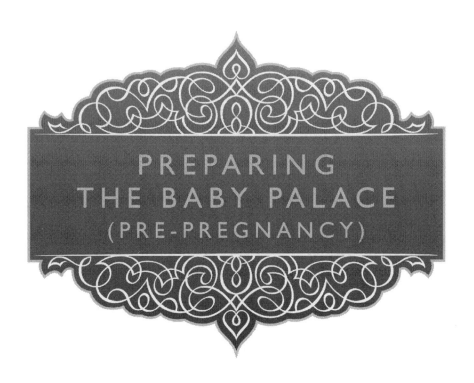

PREPARING
THE BABY PALACE
(PRE-PREGNANCY)

Making the decision to have a child is momentous. It is to decide forever to have your heart go walking around outside your body.

- Elizabeth Stone

Before deciding to have a baby for the first time, I was already meticulous about my health and fitness. With a tendency to be organized and to plan everything down to the smallest detail, baby-making would be a piece of cake—or so I thought. To my dismay, I was wrong.

What did I miss?

I followed all the rules.

Why am I not pregnant yet?

I remember scouring the web and flipping through all of my pregnancy books, desperate to find the answers. I stumbled upon the website of a local healing arts center for women. There was a service they were offering called Maya Abdominal Massage for Women's Health (The Arvigo Techniques of Abdominal Massage™), which is a non-invasive healing technique that can be used to enhance fertility. I booked an appointment right away.

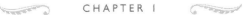

I met with Lisa, the owner, for my abdominal massage. She looked puzzled when I expressed my concern that something might be wrong with me.

"You've been trying to get pregnant for only two months; that's why you're here?"

"Er…um…yes."

"Things take time, Shivani. Relax. Stressing about it won't help at all," Lisa reassured me.

Many times in my life when I'm feeling distressed, it's the confluence of too many fear-based thoughts clouding my mind with, *Am I enough? If I don't do this, who am I?*

Before I left, Lisa recommended I read a book by Walter Makichen called *Spirit Babies: How to Communicate with the Child You're Meant to Have.* That whole exchange opened me up to the spiritual aspect of pregnancy, which is a vital component of *The Conscious Pregnancy*.

BECOME A BLANK CANVAS

Even with pregnancy, we can get caught up in playing the dreaded comparison game. I did not conceive a baby in two months, so I immediately thought I might be infertile. In reality, I was setting an unrealistic expectation for myself. Had I stopped concerning myself with the success stories of pregnant women, I may have not panicked as much as I did.

If the most important thing is this new life we are creating inside us, we've got to stop worrying about the Joneses. Let go of who you think you have to be and embrace who you are becoming — right here right now.

Think about this for a minute.

You will never again be the person you once were. You will become a mother and a creator—the center of someone's universe. You are opening up your body, mind, and spirit to create this new soul growing inside you. This new life is starting with a blank slate. He or she is relying on you to nurture him or her in your womb for the next nine to ten months and to be loved by you for the rest of your life.

Pregnancy also allows you to start over. Become a blank canvas. How you choose to paint this canvas will make all the difference in the world for your future baby and for your own livelihood. Like that elective class you took in college or noon-hour recess when you were a kid, pregnancy is a good time to take a break and to do what brings you joy. Have fun with this special time. Play.

I attended childbirth classes at the hospital and also took advantage of the education they were offering at my birthing center. I wanted a broad perspective to help prepare me for childbirth. The prenatal yoga classes were wonderful for stretching my body, easing pregnancy aches and pains, and re-centering me every week. The HypnoBirthing® class I took at the birthing center opened my eyes to new viewpoints and possibilities.

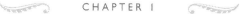

I felt myself expanding from the inside and out, which is why I regularly frequented birthing classes during pregnancy. What shocked me, however, was the resistance I received from many people who thought I was crazy for wanting to spend so much time with other pregnant organic women every Saturday.

Can I blame them?

Many of us go through life believing what we see is what we get. In mainstream culture, we're taught to fear things that deviate from the norm. We've attached stigmas to philosophies we don't quite understand. We've learned to dismiss anything that reeks of mysticism because esoteric practices are just too *woo-woo*.

When the dichotomy between Western and Eastern views on health surfaced again, I realized our world was in need of a colossal wake-up call. I know I'm not the first to have this revelation.

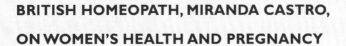

BRITISH HOMEOPATH, MIRANDA CASTRO, ON WOMEN'S HEALTH AND PREGNANCY

If you are looking to enhance your general health and well-being, yoga is my number one recommendation. Any kind of strength and flexibility you want during pregnancy, you will get from yoga. Many women take to their couches during pregnancies, which does not make logical sense because childbirth is a marathon (some are like a 10K).

In addition to staying physically fit, which is most crucial during pregnancy, nutrition is also important. Work on keeping your blood sugar levels stable. If you get crazy cravings, do your best to balance them out in some way. I was voraciously hungry during pregnancy. I put on a ridiculous amount of weight, but that reflected the stress I was under. I had self-medicated with food to handle the stress. I did not have a sensible person advising me. The books I had been reading at the time basically advised that you could do anything when you are pregnant. The acupuncture teacher I had studied under even told me, "Women give birth behind bushes all the time; it is no problem."

Listen to your fears and worries. Find someone to help you understand the message. I wish I had that perspective when I was pregnant.

This is not an attempt to ask you to reject Western practices, or to suggest that either view is evil or wrong. Gone are the days of listening to everyone else besides yourself. Whether you consider yourself a *hippie* or side with conventional practices, there are many great aspects to the spiritual undertones of the East and the science-based influences of the West. We can benefit from respecting a hybrid approach; women are looking for this balance during pregnancy.

If we want to grow, we must open ourselves up to what else exists beyond our current state of consciousness. It is possible to unlearn what we *think* we know, without abandoning our values. When we lead with curiosity and compassion, there is little to fear of the unknown. Are you tired of straddling the line between these two stereotypes as I am? Let's close the vast rift between these two worlds.

STRIVE TO BE A GOOD STEWARD OF YOUR HEALTH

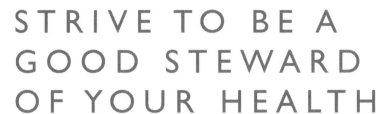

The world is full of toxins; that is a fact. Sadly, many companies are not telling you the truth about what they're putting in their products and our children are paying the price for it. Many products targeting women, such as creams and fragrances, have some of the highest levels of toxicity in their ingredients. I say this to inform you, not to instill fear in you.

Do a gradual detox well before getting pregnant. Before you conceive, give yourself time to investigate products that are safe for you and your body. Then, do a gradual detox with the resources that make the most sense to you. As with anything, uninformed or impulsive decisions may yield immediate results, but not a sustainable success.

One year before I got pregnant, I went to India for a three-week detox. I did a complete organic juice fast. My daily routine consisted of walking, yoga, and several detoxifying procedures (enemas, colonics, massages, and treatments). It was intense and also incredible. I cleansed my body in ways I would find difficulty achieving where I live in the United States.

Fortunately, you can do a similar detox as I did without having to go to India. I did a complete Ayurvedic detox called Panchakarma. Ayurveda teaches that doing Panchakarma annually can ward off any chronic disease.

Experiment with supplements before getting pregnant. Pre-pregnancy is the best phase in which to experiment with supplements for use in your detoxification programs. It is also an ideal time to eliminate lifestyle choices that could potentially sabotage a successful pregnancy.

Say you've spent the last few years smoking, drinking, eating fast food, heavily caffeinated, overworking, and underexercising. If you were to get pregnant tomorrow, you'd likely try to eliminate all of these habits immediately. Any drastic lifestyle change can have ramifications. You could become depleted of the vitamins, nutrients, and minerals keeping your body robust.

Just like an aircraft needs a runway to take flight, you will need time and space to prepare your mind, body, and spirit for pregnancy and childbirth.

Science has proven that taking a prenatal vitamin three months *before* conception is imperative for maintaining vitality during pregnancy, and reducing the risk of defects or low-weight for your child at birth. Consult your practitioner to help you identify where your vitamin and mineral levels are deficient, or in excess, so you can get back to ideal levels before conception.

I thank my lucky stars I followed this advice before I conceived. Long before I got pregnant, I found out I was Vitamin D deficient. My practitioner prescribed me 50 times the recommended daily dosage until my Vitamin D levels returned to normal.

Had I waited to consult a practitioner until after finding out I was pregnant, the high dosage level would have been unsafe to consume and, therefore, unprescribable—this would have left me Vitamin D deficient for my entire pregnancy and breastfeeding years (which can be up to two years!).

Can you imagine you and your baby being without the proper nutrients for up to two years?

Check the toxicity level of products in your home. We are fortunate we live in a time where there is now data available to research the ingredients companies have been putting into skin care products over the last century. Those ingredients, which have been entirely experimental, include Bisphenol A (BPA), and many toxic substances that are on lists of known carcinogens—substances that cause cancer.

As I write this, scientific studies are revealing Bisphenol S (BPS), which is what manufacturers switched to from BPA, can be just as toxic as BPA. This knowledge alone may not sway us to stop using all of these toxic products at once, since we're now told that almost everything on Earth can cause cancer.

Getting rid of toxins from your environment is a simple concept, but not an easy task. Transforming your environment will be a process; it will take time. If you've been waiting to revamp your beauty cabinet and cleaning closet, becoming pregnant offers an excellent opportunity to do so.

As you clean your home and get the nursery ready for the baby, it is especially vital that you also prepare your baby palace. The term *baby palace* is a concept from acupuncture (an ancient Chinese healing modality). Acupuncture has a philosophy that believes every seed needs healthy soil to grow—just as every embryo needs a healthy womb to nurture it to become a fetus.

The primary goal during pregnancy is to create a full and nutrient-rich uterine lining to support the growth of a new baby. That being said, you do not want any crazy chemicals interacting with or floating inside the baby palace. Studies have shown that the blood in the umbilical cord of a baby at birth—in many women—has a higher concentration of BPA than what we consider safe levels in the United States. Some fetuses are feeding off of a host of chemicals (more chemicals than are safe for an adult!) that can damage his or her health. Unfortunately, since our bodies cannot detect whether substances are foreign, this means toxins can accumulate in different places in the body and manifest as disease.

Thyroid problems and autoimmune disorders (where our immune systems are attacking healthy cells) have become epidemics, a fact which unnerves me to no end. If these problems could be perpetuated by the toxic ingredients used to manufacture and package our skincare or cleaning products (or even the food we consume), wouldn't you want to equip yourself with this information so you can take precaution?

Support environmentally conscious companies. Fueled by the knowledge we're gaining in this society, we have become powerful human search engines. We are able to identify which of the big brands out there—some of which we've known and loved for decades — are built by companies that (intentionally or inadvertently) have been compromising our safety. Many of these businesses have concerned themselves with shelf stability, reducing costs, and improving aesthetics or aroma at the expense of our long-term health.

We, the consumers, have demanded safer products for the environment, for our bodies, and for our babies. In this modern age, we are witnessing an influx of environmentally conscious companies that are stepping up. Many of these new companies — created by mothers and fathers who also wanted a better solution for their own children — are challenging themselves to find a better way to do things.

If we wish to create a safer environment for our children, we must support environmentally conscious companies by voting with our dollars and voices.

Do your best every day. You don't have to deprive yourself to live a less toxic life. You can challenge the status quo. You can become a good steward of your own health. Success may not happen overnight, but you will be able to reduce the total toxic burden on your body and protect your unborn child if you do your best every day.

This whole premise is why I started *Sama Baby Organics* in 2006. At the time, organic clothing for children was rough, ugly, and uncomfortable. Parents wanted premium quality for their babies, but not at the cost of comfort and well-being. I saw this gap in the market and I knew there had to be a better way. That entrepreneurial journey took me to India where I researched cotton farmers, factories, international standards for non-toxic dyes, and fashion. I co-launched a beautiful line of clothing that moms not only loved, but needed.

Do you have to start an organic clothing line to lead a less toxic life? No. You can become an informed consumer by becoming a better student.

First, you can identify which products contain toxic chemicals, carcinogens, BPA, and preservatives. Then, your research can inform your decisions about which products to remove and replace with less toxic ones. Little by little, these deliberate choices you make can become ingrained in your daily routine.

Challenge what you think you already know. Question the dogma fed to you. Make your choice based on your beliefs and values—not because of popularity. Avoid the fads. You are a conduit for love to move through you. Trust your intuition. The conscious awakening is already happening as you read these words. Own your power and do your best every day.

Here are some questions that can help you explore the current state of your health and lifestyle:

THE CONSCIOUS PREGNANCY LIFESTYLE SELF-SURVEY

Am I eating a balanced and nutritious diet?

Am I engaging in physical activity daily?

Am I getting enough sleep?

Do I minimize my exposure to environmental toxins?

Do I avoid any harmful drugs or toxic products that could endanger my body and my future baby?

Do I recycle or find ways to not create excessive waste?

Do I change my air filters as recommended?

Am I managing my stress levels at work?

Where you answered "yes" to any of the questions in the self-survey, great job! Keep it up.

If you answered "no" to any of the questions, I've included some simple rituals for self-care at the end of this chapter.

In the back of this book, you'll also find a resource guide ("Appendix A: The Conscious Pregnancy Lifestyle Choices") to help you get started on ways to improve your lifestyle.

Set Aside Time and Space for Self-Care

Before you conceive, explore spiritual rituals that help you quiet your mind and prepare your body for the exquisite experience of creating new life. The consequences are too damaging for the future baby if we neglect self-care—especially before becoming pregnant.

I learned quickly during my first pregnancy that reacting to the happenings of my busy world was negatively affecting me. Although I hadn't yet become a mom, at the time, I realized I had the power to be a mother warrior and protect this tiny seed I would grow inside me.

Unfortunately, I would have to find this out the hard way.

Slow down and take care of yourself. When I discovered I was pregnant, I continued with my rigorous workouts. I kept running from one client meeting to another, as the owner of my boutique PR firm. My usual routine would be short-lived because my CEO lifestyle was not conducive to a pregnant one. It was difficult turning off this wiring because old habits die hard.

My obstetrician instructed me I could continue with my workout regimen as long as my maximum heart rate was 140. This drove me nuts! I did spin class and lifted weights three times per week before I conceived just so I could continue this regimen during my pregnancy (hoping it would help me quickly bounce back to my fit and awesome pre-pregnancy physique).

As my doctor warned, I did end up significantly modifying my workout regimen to accommodate this rule because my heart rate would always exceed 140.

"Can I be exempt from this rule?" I asked my obstetrician.

"Sure, you can work out that way for an hour. Just hold your breath the whole time."

It turns out that the equivalent of continuing at that intensity level of my rigorous workout regimen would mean depriving my baby of oxygen for the entire hour. It wasn't worth it.

Do you have to be headstanding yogi on the beach or a spin ninja in the gym? No. Despite what the media depicts as healthy living, rigorous workouts at the gym or yoga headstands on the beach can both be stress-inducing activities—if the goal is striving for sheer perfection and flawless beauty.

Stress causes inflammation, which is known to be linked to chronic disease and cancer. Therefore, the goal of reaching perfection or optimal health is actually counterproductive.

We must do things in moderation. I had a hard time with this being quite the overachiever. But, I learned to schedule daily cues and reminders to help me prioritize self-care, which improved my energy immensely. The self-care activities I chose included visiting an Ayurvedic practitioner, joining a yoga class, meditating on my own, and scheduling a two-hour time block to create space for peace and quiet (listening to relaxing music in bed or taking a nap).

Whatever you choose, make sure to take advantage of the expansive creativity and stillness your consciousness craves during pregnancy, especially if you want to create a future Zen Baby. Remember, the choices you make in the six months to a year before you conceive will be key to achieving a conscious pregnancy and future Zen Baby.

Here are some of the subtlest ways you can slow down and make time for self-care rituals every day:

SIMPLE SELF-CARE RITUALS

- Find a prenatal yoga studio nearby (yoga stretches your muscles, ligaments, and body) to enjoy a more blissful state of being.
- Can't make it to a prenatal yoga studio? Take a shower, pull out your yoga mat, and stretch.
- Set a daily a mantra or positive intention before you leave the house.
- Put on jewelry or semi-precious stones that balance or enhance your energy.
- Listen to a peaceful CD with sweet and touching affirmations. Or, listen to an inspiring audio book that uplifts you on your drive home.

- Watch a movie or TV program (nothing violent or disruptive) in the evening with your partner.

- Treat yourself to a decadent dinner.

- Take a walk out in nature.

- Take vitamin D and any other supplements that support your pregnancy.

- Bathe with your favorite essential oils and add salt or flower petals.

- Light a candle.

- Spend a few moments in positive thought, saying a prayer, or meditating before bed.

- Journal to get your thoughts out of your head and feelings out of your heart.

- Keep a gratitude log; write five things you're grateful for daily.

At the end of this book, I share additional resources you can apply immediately to begin making shifts in your lifestyle (see "Appendix A: The Conscious Pregnancy Lifestyle Choices") and to your nutrition (see "Appendix B: The Conscious Pregnancy Diet Guidelines") to support your baby-making efforts.

The Sad, Sick & Spent Phase

CHAPTER 2:

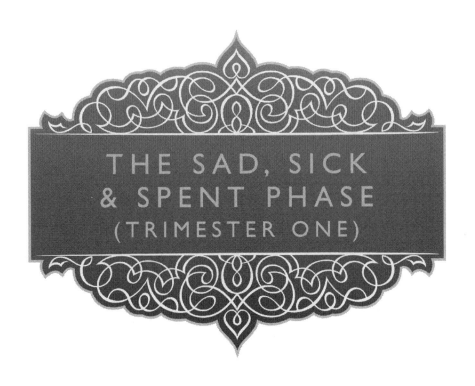

THE SAD, SICK
& SPENT PHASE
(TRIMESTER ONE)

Experience is determined by yourself — not the circumstances of your life. - Gita Bellin

By now, you may be drowning in the bottomless pit of articles and advertisements bombarding you on *how to have a healthy and happy pregnancy* by eating this, doing this, and not doing that. How can you possibly implement everything you read in books or watch on TV? Where would you even start? There's so much to do and so little time. No wonder we can feel overwhelmed in the first trimester, which I call *The Sad, Sick, and Spent Phase.*

During pregnancy, your hormones are raging. Your body makes significant physical changes. The emotions you feel — anger, happiness, joy, resentment — are also felt by your unborn baby. For this reason, pregnancy can be a recipe for disaster at times. Therefore, it is increasingly important that you practice self-care.

For the Type A mom who wants everything 100 percent perfect for her pregnancy, this message is especially for you (trust me, I am that mom!). We obsess about what is best for our home, for our body, for our family, and for our environment. There's one little problem with obsessing: we're driving ourselves (and everyone around us) crazy as we end up running on empty by trying to be everything to everyone all the time.

There is no connection more powerful than a mother's love — first for herself and, then, for the new life she will create. Self-care is taking pause to *be* healthy and happy in your pregnancy — not obsess about it.

While I was pregnant with my first child, I remember waking up and finding red stretch marks all over my belly — it horrified me.

"It's going to be okay, that's a natural part of pregnancy. Don't worry, they will go away," my husband reassured me.

Every night, he helped me rub coconut oil over my stretch marks. It was such a mortifying experience because the perfectionist in me was doubtful my soft, supple skin would ever return.

Pregnancy is real. You'll get real symptoms and real, uncomfortable experiences. You'll also make real sacrifices. People rarely talk about the psychological impact pregnancy has on women. Hundreds of years ago (even decades ago) having children was the primary role of a woman. A woman's job was to marry young and make babies. Personal beauty, career, self-development—these were not priorities for women.

It is a vastly different time we live in now. We, as a people, are becoming more individualized. We, as women, are now focusing on our own well-being, career, and personal aspirations in addition to our childbearing duties. Today, we seem to have a very different problem on our hands. Experiences that were once cherished are becoming transactional, emotionless, and uneventful.

Nobody ever says, "I want to have an unhappy pregnancy and unhealthy baby." We're just busy. We have a hectic schedule and a long to-do list—I get it. Whether we've witnessed other women who have become jaded and unexcited about pregnancy or we've been taught to feel it's a burden a woman has to go through to make a child, we're now commoditizing pregnancy—just as we do with everything else we juggle in our lives.

I will not sugar coat pregnancy for you: that nine-month period can be unbearable at times. You get large. You feel uncomfortable. You put up with a lot of pain. Your brain gets foggy. You become vulnerable and dependent on others. Some may describe it as an irritation and an injustice just to get the results you want: a baby. But it doesn't have to make you feel this way!

As you read in the previous chapter, self-care is one of the most unselfish acts you can do for your body before becoming pregnant. It is also important for you to prioritize the time, space, and energy that you'll need for taking care of your emotional well-being during pregnancy. When you do this, you connect to a higher vibrational frequency that can manifest as love and nurturing for you and the fetus growing inside your womb.

Practicing Indulgence Daily

Few people have healthy outlets for the loud, busy, stressful, and draining lives we lead. That's why we turn to overeating, overdrinking, and binging. That's why we distract ourselves with social media and TV. There are more productive ways to cope.

There may be periods of time you will want to lie down and do nothing during pregnancy. Relish those peaceful moments. Bask in the stillness and appreciate the benefits that come with honoring the needs of your womb—the ultimate vessel of health for your future Zen Baby.

Whether you define yourself as religious or spiritual, there is a ritualistic aspect to either practice. The rosary, mala, lighting of candles, unique treasures or offerings in front of the symbol of the god or leader—these are all rituals. The practice of bathing yourself, brushing your teeth, getting dressed, and feeding your family are also rituals. Rituals are a powerful way to create a peaceful haven for yourself, in your home, and for your spiritual practice. Which kind of rituals help you feel happy, centered and balanced? Do more of them, especially in *The Sad, Sick, and Spent Phase.*

Create sacred spaces in your home to help you achieve these rituals: a special place to sit and drink tea, an altar with your cues for meditation, a shelf in the bathroom full of oils and creams to pamper yourself. Work full time? There are ways to sneak in small self-care rituals in your workday. For example, I run my business from my home, which means I can go to my sacred shelf in the bathroom to put on lotion even while I'm on a conference call. Set up your sacred space to support the flow of your routine and home.

According to Ayurveda, the daily morning routine is a cornerstone of a healthy life. All fifteen steps of this routine are a healthy component to starting your morning. The benefits: a lubricated and energized body, a sharp and clear mind, and the ability to take on your day in optimal shape.

Let's say you're a modern woman with a 40 to 50-hour a week job. You're rushing in the morning…throwing business clothes on…shoving instant breakfast down your throat…feeling ambivalent about the way you look in the mirror. You hustle hard all day at work. After work, you rush home and pick up take-out just in time for dinner with the family. It's 10:00 PM by the time you're done with the day's activities and household chores. By now, you're ready to pass out and go to sleep. Sound like you?

Now, imagine a new ritual. You're pregnant and you work no more than 40 hours a week. You do a daily Ayurvedic massage in the morning. You slather your body with organic coconut oil to nourish your skin. Not only does this calm you, but it also makes your skin glow. After a productive day at work, you take five minutes to anoint your body with oil. Before bedtime, you write in your gratitude journal. You're happier because you did something for yourself to fuel your soul, instead of reacting to the beat of the day.

All of these positive emotions in this new ritual are excellent ways to set intentions each morning when you wake and every night when you go to bed. Equally important, these emotions wash over the baby growing inside you.

Now, I know this may sound ethereal for you to read. Knowledge is only powerful if you're doing something with the strategies and tools you learn. Experiment. Apply what you learn. You must practice a new activity consistently before you can turn it into a habit—that goes for the good and bad ones.

The Sad, Sick, and Spent Phase is about accepting the changes to come. Your life will evolve in ways you've never imagined before. If you haven't already implemented a framework to support yourself, now is the time to make that conscious choice.

Create space for ritualistic activities that help you slow down, and stay centered and balanced for the next nine to ten months. The following list contains Ayurvedic must do's you can implement during pregnancy:

AYURVEDIC MUST DO'S

- Avoid physical labor, fasting, or activities that emaciate the body or cause it grief and fright. Avoid scary TV shows, books. Also, the news can be detrimental because it could cause jerky movements.
- Avoid eating dry, stale, or old food from the previous day.
- Avoid synthetic or strong perfumes and oils.
- Avoid going to the extreme or doing anything in excess. Too much sour, salty, sweet, bitter, spicy, astringent, or pungent things can aggravate you.

- Reconsider getting into quarrels, fights, adding grief, or thinking ill of others as these can lead to adverse outcomes for your future child.
- Be joyful.
- Wear clean white garments or light colored clothes.
- Engage in peace-giving activities.
- Follow a month-by-month diet of what to include in the pregnancy for a healthy baby.
- Read religious books, spiritual books or books of higher thinking; all of this knowledge passes on to the child.

To access a summary of the Ideal Ayurvedic Morning Routine, visit the book resources page at The ConsciousPregnancy.com.

Taking a Proactive Approach

As I alluded to earlier, I was obsessive during my first pregnancy. Everything had to be just right and in its place. I'll never forget the time I was seven months pregnant and standing on a ladder organizing all of the cans so the labels lined up. I had stocked up my shelves as if Hurricane Shivani was on the horizon. I mistakenly believed I would never leave the house after the baby arrived, so I convinced myself I had to prepare accordingly. In hindsight, I know I had put myself at risk for something that gave me only two seconds of satisfaction.

I spent most of that pregnancy wasting precious energy on trivial things that did not benefit my health. I refused to trust anyone to help me clean or prepare the nursery. I dealt with a lot of insomnia and gained a lot of weight for my small frame. I felt uncomfortable, had limited mobility, and my stress levels were through the roof. I filled myself with junk food to cope. I spiraled out of control in order to remain in control. It was exhausting and ultimately not worth it.

I know my story is not unique; neither is yours.

We live in a reactionary world. A lot is going on in the environment. When we choose to react to these internal and external pressures instead of taking a proactive approach, we disconnect from our own truth. You don't have to cower underneath your blanket for the next nine or ten months feeling defeated by fear-mongering advice. You can treat pregnancy like the sacred and special time that it is.

I'd be remiss if I failed to mention the basics of what to do when you find out you're pregnant:

BASIC MUST DO'S

- Find a practitioner: midwife or obstetrician. Shop around, interview, and ask for referrals. Choose someone whose belief system resonates with yours. Do not settle.
- Find a birthing center or hospital that aligns with your views and values.
- Find a doula, a HypnoBirthing® class, a sacred pregnancy class, a prenatal yoga class, or other means of spiritual education and coaching.
- Take your prenatal vitamins regularly: fish oil and any other supplements you need.

- Eat a balanced, nutritious diet, and cut out the bad stuff.

- Eliminate alcohol, smoking, heavy lifting, excessive exercise, and fasting.

- Stay active. Walking and yoga are excellent. Consult your practitioner with any questions you have about other activities to explore.

Being proactive is acknowledging that the growing fetus inside you is full of promise and hope. He or she is capable of achieving mental, spiritual, and physical greatness if you choose to listen to your body and trust that you intuitively know what is right for you.

For additional resources, see "Appendix D: Terms, Definitions, and Resources from the Experts" in the back of this book.

The Beautiful, Blessed, & Blissful Phase

CHAPTER 3:

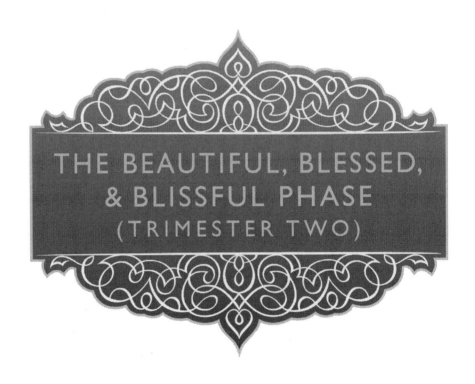

THE BEAUTIFUL, BLESSED,
& BLISSFUL PHASE
(TRIMESTER TWO)

Courage is like a muscle. We strengthen it with use. - Ruth Gordon

In *The Sad, Sick, and Spent Phase*, I encouraged you to make immediate changes in your lifestyle and environment once you knew you were pregnant. By changes, I'm talking about subtle changes. Depriving yourself of everything or doing a complete overhaul of your life can have adverse effects if not done in moderation.

Moderation is the Key

Do things in moderation early on because it will set the tone for the rest of your pregnancy. After learning I was pregnant, I eliminated anything that would directly harm my unborn baby. As with everything else, I modified what I could from my daily routine.

I continued to do the same exercises as I did before, as I mentioned earlier, but I reduced the intensity level to give my body a break since it was changing. If I ever found myself in a stressful situation, I'd create a bubble I could retreat to. Naturally, you want to avoid a loud bar or party that overstimulates your energy during pregnancy. If it's challenging to control the noise, the heat, or the people around you, having the bubble helps you check out from the rest of the world.

Never subject yourself to the discomfort, it will only aggravate you — especially as your body expands. I also used the bubble to escape emotionally from my environment. If I ever felt negatively affected by others, I'd retreat into my bubble to prevent their words and actions from provoking me to feel unhappy or potentially harming the baby.

Find peace however you see fit. You can chant mantras in your head, or hum a tune that calms and relaxes you. If I was unable to get to my music, I would imagine myself lying listening to peaceful tunes in a cool, comfortable bed. As you may know, the brain can't decipher between something you're visualizing and something that's actually happening, but it will produce the same feelings associated with the thought or emotion (real or imagined).

In Ayurvedic and ancient traditions in India, a pregnant woman is not allowed to watch violent TV shows or movies, listen to loud or angry music, attend funerals and sad occasions, or learn of anything that has happened to a pregnant woman or new mom. Since the mother's mental state is so closely guarded by those around her, it is essential that she create a bubble to shield herself from negative energy. Our ancestors innately knew that what the mother feels, the baby also feels. Today, this belief holds true.

Charaka, the Father of Ayurveda, wrote a text around 400 BCE called Charaka Samhita — the most important ancient authoritative writings on Ayurveda. According to Charaka Samhita, pregnant women who follow the Ayurvedic recommendations will give birth to a desired, famous, long-living, and healthy baby. A woman who desires excellent progeny must particularly refrain from unwholesome diet and behavior. Ancient scriptures tell stories of mothers who, after reading religious books or singing religious songs every day to their unborn children, gave birth to babies with the knowledge of a priest or wise man. Who wouldn't want excellent offspring, right? Well, it's easier said than done in our modern times.

If the mind has the power to create a sanctuary when we need to protect ourselves from harmful emotions, that means we also have the ability to protect the little one growing inside us before he or she is even born.

Choose to fill your time with spiritual or religious knowledge. Read things that fill your cup. Listen to classical or peaceful music. Take an hour to lie in bed and rest. Allow yourself to drift into deep relaxation. If you choose to consciously retreat like this at any point of the day, silence your phone, close your door, and shut out the outside world.

Consider this moment as your time to simply *be*. You can do this for fifteen minutes, one hour, or longer if you can prioritize the time. You can also use a meditation app if that helps you to achieve stillness.

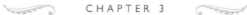
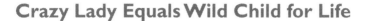

Crazy Lady Equals Wild Child for Life

Scientists have uncovered a significant relationship between our lifestyles and the onset of disease. The science is irrefutable, especially regarding cancer and other life-threatening chronic illnesses. We have the power to influence many of the positive health outcomes that we all want.

Adopting a healthy lifestyle before deciding to have a baby, and maintaining that type of regimen post-pregnancy, can make a significant impact on the pregnancy and childbirth process.

The logic is simple. If an activity can harm our health or the environment, we must take precaution. Our body gives us indicators to help us decipher whether a choice we make makes us feel good or not. During pregnancy, for example, women have a very keen sense of sound and smell. One poignant example of this that I recall during my pregnancy came when I was standing with my husband outside of an airport and breathing secondhand smoke. Instead of being slightly repulsed by the smell as I usually would be, I felt an immense urge to run in the other direction. My husband told me I was overreacting. His senses were obviously not as heightened as mine. I say this not to be facetious; it's the truth.

If something smells bad, your senses are warning you to get out of there—a bad chemical may have been used there! Use this heightened skill to your advantage during pregnancy—there is no room to grin and bear it.

A pregnant mom knows best. Trust your maternal instincts. Flex your mama bear muscles. Do not acquiesce to people of authority, people in your family, or people you might inherently hold in high regard. Otherwise, you and your unborn child may end up paying the price for going with politeness instead of intuition.

Many pregnant women have also found themselves suddenly becoming disgusted by foods they previously craved. This goes both ways. Follow your intuition. Your body innately knows what it does and does not need. Avoid anything that you find intolerable (taste or smell). Whenever in doubt, we must err on the side of caution. It is not worth putting yourself or your unborn baby at risk.

It's crucial to routinely assess how you treat yourself and your body, especially as you move further along in the pregnancy. Do you often say no to yourself? Do you deny yourself of activities that will benefit your health? For example, do you stay up late working to finish a work deadline even though you know your mind and body need a break? Or, are you operating at the same capacity at five months pregnant that you were at three months? Now is the time to change this behavior, if you haven't started already.

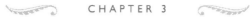

The price of a crazy woman during pregnancy is a wild child for life! If we could realize the power we hold to make hell or heaven out of any given situation (pregnant or not), we would be happier and healthier human beings. There is no question we have the ability to remove ourselves from stressful situations. It just requires that we become better gatekeepers of our minds. This will require a lot of practice and patience, but we alone have the power to control what we are letting in and out of the gate. We can whip that little monkey into submission.

How do you succeed as a new mom without neglecting any other area of your life? The balance you seek is possible, but improbable at the same time.

In the United States, the importance of measuring results is deeply engrained in society. We, modern women, have a lot going on and yet so much to prove — to achieve. We strive to be superwomen — triple threats — beautiful, smart, and successful. We feel must be everything all at once and all of the time.

What pregnancy, childbirth, and raising children all teach us is that we put way too much pressure on ourselves to achieve unrealistic ideals — I've experienced the struggle firsthand and witnessed many women who've also dealt with this self-sabotage. We ask ourselves, *Why can't I have it all? Look at Gisele Bunche. She's an organic mom with gorgeous hair, a hot body, successful career, sexy husband, beautiful babies, and a green lifestyle! If she can do it all, I should be able to do it all too.*

At some point in our lives, we have driven ourselves crazy with unrealistic expectations we've set for our lives. Let's say you get pretty darn close to perfection. Once achieved, could you sustain that level of happiness all the time? Are you willing to sacrifice magical moments with these joyful beings you birthed to get it?

It is rarely those airbrushed and photoshopped moments in life that resonate with us when we look back at in time. For me, I find happiness in the simple moments of my life: rolling around with the kids on the family room floor, reminiscing with my husband right before bed, and taking my family out to our favorite local diner on the weekend. Few of us have nutritionists, trainers, chefs, assistants and personal drivers supporting our lifestyle as celebrities do.

Release the façade of being Supermom and you'll free your soul. Master the balancing act of the ebb and flow of life and you will master motherhood.

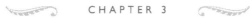

I refer to the second trimester as *The Beautiful, Blessed, and Blissful Phase* not because you will be free of stress, distractions or interruptions. In the second trimester, you have the option of retreating to your bubble and turning things around in spite of the craziness that pregnancy can bring.

Multi-tasking, though natural for women, must be avoided or at least reduced during pregnancy. Do one thing at a time. You can meet the demands of being the mother and caretaker of your family without compromising your sanity. Playing peaceful music (I listen to Jai Uttal from my prenatal yoga days) can help relax the mood. My favorite radio stations on Pandora are Spa Music, Yoga Music, Snatam Kaur, The Piano Guys, and Coldplay.

Surviving Pregnancy Fog

Your body has a mind of its own when you're pregnant because it has decided the fetus is the top priority. Fortunately and unfortunately, it is like a diversion of resources.

Think of yourself as a full cup before getting pregnant. After conception, it is no surprise when you start forgetting where you left your keys or parked your car. Pregnancy fog is what this phenomenon is called, and it really does exist. Your body is shifting. Your hormones and blood flow are changing to orient your body for the creation of a baby. Your body's energy is diverted to support the immense undertaking of nurturing the growing fetus inside of you. Instead of being at full capacity, you're operating at 90 percent or less during pregnancy.

With each trimester, your mind may become foggier. Allow space for these changes to occur. Fighting against them is fighting against nature and that is futile. If you accept this notion, you accept that you may be less capable of accomplishing things the way you used to as time progresses.

Realize that on any given day, you will be able to do some things and unable to do others. You will have good days and bad. Leave space for openness, consciousness, and creativity. Build messiness and unexpected moments into your routine—they end up creating some of the most beautiful memories.

I have instituted a 20 percent rule, which means that I accept that 20 percent of my day will inevitably change. This expectation provides for the fact that I must allow for time to accommodate unforeseen circumstances.

When I was pregnant, there were many times when someone would call me with something urgent and ask for my help, but because I had allotted time for cases where I might have needed to cancel things last minute, reschedule or move things around I was able to handle these unexpected events with ease. I encourage you to build a cushion of flexibility into your day to help mitigate stress.

The third trimester is also a good time to tell your spouse, partner, and family that you will likely soon need their help. Get the crazy idea out of your mind that you have to do it all—your body will simply not allow it. Motherhood is one long chain of unexpected occurrences. Train those around you to pitch in, take over responsibilities, and lighten your load. Asking for help is another means of self-care.

Decrease the intensity level of your activities, but also, move your body in this phase. Moving reduces how sluggish you'll feel as your belly grows. Trying is not the same thing as doing. I recently found myself dreading the thought of going to the gym. As active as I am, I hate going to a gym to work out. I reached a point where I kept saying I would go, but came up with every excuse not to (now that I'm a busy mom of two). *I'll try going to the gym tomorrow,* I told myself.

I recognized that saying I'll *try* something instead of actually *doing* it gave me permission to not commit to making it happen. What bothers me most is when I am out of integrity with my words and actions. I stopped what I was doing that day and I *went* to the gym. It might sound silly that I only stayed at the gym for five minutes, but I did what I set out to do — I went to the gym and moved my body.

Will we at times forget to do what's best for us? Of course. The mind can be a tricky thing when you have pregnancy fog. Remember, the negative messages you send to your unborn baby can manifest as unwanted behaviors or diseases. Nurture your child before you give birth. If you want your baby to be calm, you have to be peaceful. Create a healthy and loving sanctuary for yourself and your growing fetus.

Being pregnant is an excellent time to slow down and get in touch with your creative side. I surveyed a handful of women while writing this book. Most of them said they did not think of pregnancy as a time to be creative. I was fortunate to have friends who painted a lot when they were pregnant; I saw firsthand how it opened them up creatively.

Whether you consider yourself artistic or not, these types of creative activities and exercises open you up to a world of possibility and creation. Exercising is not only for the physical body. Through creative expression, you are also stimulating your brain. Imagine what your creative energy can do for your happiness, your peace, and your baby's well-being when you explore this part of yourself.

Though you may be physically limited or restricted in some ways, see this time as an opportunity to engage in activities you would rarely make time for. Sign up for that painting class that you have been eyeing for years!

I was an active patron of my birthing center where I was encouraged to make all sorts of crafts, including paintings, necklaces, and cards — things I've always wanted to do but often found excuses not to.

Looking for ways to explore your creativity? Check out this list for ideas to get your creative juices flowing:

WAYS TO CHANNEL YOUR CREATIVE ENERGIES

- Do a pregnancy art project.
- Paint items for the nursery.
- Sew, knit, crochet, and craft things for your home or nursery.
- Journal, write, express everything going on in your mind.
- Bake bread from scratch or something else you might be craving.
- Go to a butterfly museum, botanical garden, or arboretum.
- Sketch what you see.
- Read.
- Dabble in photography.
- Write.
- Listen to new music, play an instrument, or enjoy live music.
- Do things that help you to feel beautiful.
- Engage in activities that make you happy.

The Eager, Excruciating, & Equipped Phase

CHAPTER 4:

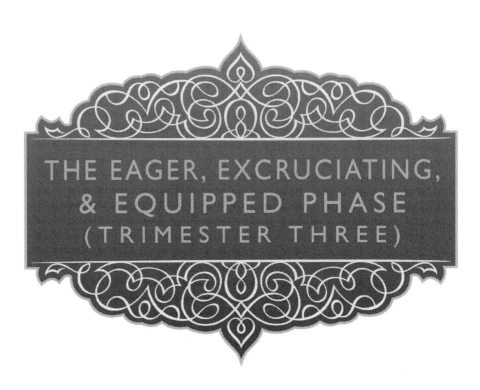

THE EAGER, EXCRUCIATING,
& EQUIPPED PHASE
(TRIMESTER THREE)

A woman is the full circle. Within her is the power to create, nurture and transform. - Diane Mariechild

As many childbirth stories have repeatedly taught us, "the more you plan, the more your plan unravels." I learned this lesson when I decided to get induced and have an epidural for my daughter's birth—all contrary to my original plans. As you read in the introduction chapter, Anya's lung had collapsed and I became disconnected from her while they kept her in the NICU for ten days.

I say this not to scare you, but rather to help you avoid the pitfalls of not allowing for flexibility in your birth plan. If you equip yourself with knowledge and resources that support your values and views on child birthing, you can make more informed choices and you can find a happy medium.

Conscious Birthing

Women have several choices for birthing their baby in this modern age. Many beautiful courses, such as HypnoBirthing®, sacred pregnancy, and prenatal yoga can guide you through the process of childbirth.

I learned something that shocked me to the core in the HypnoBirthing® class I took. In the 1960s, "Standard of Care" in hospitals stated that all births had to take place in a sterile hospital setting under the care of an obstetrician. The laboring mother is heavily sedated during childbirth. By the time the new mom comes to, her baby has already been delivered and taken to the nursery. Only after three days can the new mom can then pick up her baby from the hospital and go home.

After making this discovery, I weighed my options and revamped my child birthing plans. With my first pregnancy, I remember thinking, *No fucking hospital will dictate what I can and cannot do with a child I produced in my body and will raise under my care for the rest of my life!*

My viewpoint on giving birth in hospitals versus birthing centers or at home is quite open. It has to be. I've attended almost every kind of birth. I've wheeled a family member into her C-section appointment and slept in the recovery room with her overnight. I've also participated in a natural hospital birth where no epidural was administered. I've talked to women about their birthing stories—many of whom expressed how their choices left an imprint on their lives and left them with less than joyful experiences.

Your birthing experience will stay with you forever. If you've felt abandoned, unheard, or violated, that may frame a traumatic childbirth experience for you. If you've felt peace, love, acceptance, or nurturing at childbirth, that will shape the birthing process as a pleasant experience.

Research and interview your obstetrician, midwife, doula, or childbirth partner. Take inventory of the pros and cons of getting an epidural. Visit the hospital or birthing center you're contemplating to experience the environment and staff before making a decision. Birthing centers and many hospitals allow for water births if you're considering this option.

Do your homework to prepare accordingly for the child birthing process, but do not obsess about the location. Remember, the nine-month journey is the primary focus. Savor the journey. You will have the rest of your life to enjoy motherhood and your new child.

Ayurveda and Constipation

In the third trimester of pregnancy, *The Eager, Excruciating, and Equipped Phase,* you may be feeling more constipated. According to Ayurveda, a bowel movement a day is the key to keeping the doctor away. This topic of conversation is one that few women like to discuss. During pregnancy, constipation can become a major issue for many women.

The digestive process is a sequential downward process with many important steps, actions, and processes and the flow of this process is disrupted when you are constipated. Elimination ideally happens each morning within an hour of rising. The elimination should pass quickly, be light brown in color, and well-formed in the shape of a banana (thank you, Oprah, for bringing this health topic to the forefront!).

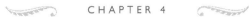

In Ayurveda, constipation is viewed as a deficiency of apana (the gradual slowing of energy responsible for excretion). Ayurveda and Western medicine both agree that occasional constipation is generally caused by too much dryness resulting from improper diet and lifestyle choices. Eating foods that are cold, dry, old, processed, and lacking in nutrients or fiber can cause constipation. Eating incompatible food combinations will also disrupt the digestive process and lead to constipation.

Other triggers of constipation include travel, drugs, supplements, illnesses, pregnancy, strain, stress, lack of physical exercise, irregular eating habits or ignoring the urge to excrete. If you have chronic or occasional constipation that bothers you, seek advice from your health care practitioner. Also, an Ayurvedic consultation can help you isolate the issue and balance your digestive system through a personalized regimen.

Back Pain, Discomfort, and Final Leg of the Journey

The Eager, Excruciating, and Equipped Phase is one of the most unique times you will ever encounter. During this phase, you will need a strong support system to lean on.

The mental discomfort and challenges you deal with in the third trimester are rare, unless you've already been pregnant before. If you make it through the final trimester without too much fuss, then you are home free.

I used to worry that bad things would happen to me during this phase.

What if my ankles are so swollen and I'm waddling too much to drive myself anywhere or be independent?

What if I'm put on bedrest and confined to nothing but TV and sleeping all day?

After having two children, I know that there are worse things than fretting about all the weight gain or feeling uncomfortable like a balloon ready to pop.

I encourage new moms to consider this thought: *If the end result is a healthy and happy baby, I can bear this discomfort a little while longer.*

Your job, at this point, is to figure out how to keep yourself spirited. You'll experience hundreds of different aches and pains. It's a challenging part of pregnancy because new issues can crop up and there are no perfect solutions. Too much of anything is never good for the baby. That goes for pain medications or any activity that can stress your emotional, mental or physical body.

Many women say that working full time makes it hard to do any of the activities prescribed for a healthy and happy pregnancy. I encourage you to start by fitting one to two of the following uplifting activities into your weekly schedule to give you a reserve of positive emotions that can help to relieve your aches and pains.

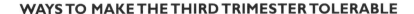
WAYS TO MAKE THE THIRD TRIMESTER TOLERABLE

- Stay mobile—walk, dance, move.
- Go to prenatal yoga, it's incredible in reducing discomfort, back pain, and other tensions.
- Soak in a tub of Epsom salt or essential oils. Relax your whole body.
- Swim (takes the weight off and helps you relax).
- Take quiet time every day to sit in a chair or lie down in bed, with peaceful music, napping or relaxing with your phone on silent.
- Meet with friends for tea, dessert, lunch, or anything to get you showered and out of the house. Connect with the people you enjoy.
- Plan for the baby. Get the final baby items ready to go: crib, clothes, nursery items, baby gear.
- Enjoy any baby showers or baby blessings. It is a beautiful time to celebrate yourself and the new baby.
- Anything you can do to make time for yourself—go to a movie, get a mani-pedi. Leaving the house will be hard with a newborn. Anything you love doing outside the house, do it before the baby arrives.

The Eager, Excruciating, and Equipped Phase is the calm before the storm. Once the baby comes, it's a flurry of activity. You'll have to figure out the baby's schedule: when to feed, sleep, bathe, or comfort your precious one —it will occupy your full time. In this final leg of your pregnancy, create boundaries because you will be starved for free time once the baby arrives.

Unlike the first two trimesters, where you are busy moving and exploring your new body and lifestyle, *The Eager, Excruciating, and Equipped Phase* is your permission slip for slowing down. Many women I've interviewed share their third-trimester scares involving blood pressure issues and trips to the ER at the very end of their pregnancies. They regret pushing past their limits.

Pregnancy is a marathon, and this is the leg of the race where you will feel the burn. You will feel the exhaustion—your motivation faltering.

Think of this guidebook as your inner cheerleader's voice. Leaf through these chapters anytime you're searching for strategies or tools to help you relax, unwind, explore, connect, align, and keep positive. If you can view your pregnancy as a magical experience with a healthy baby as the prize, the journey will be absolutely worth the twists and turns.

The Rebuilding,
Restoring,
& Renewing
Phase

CHAPTER 5:

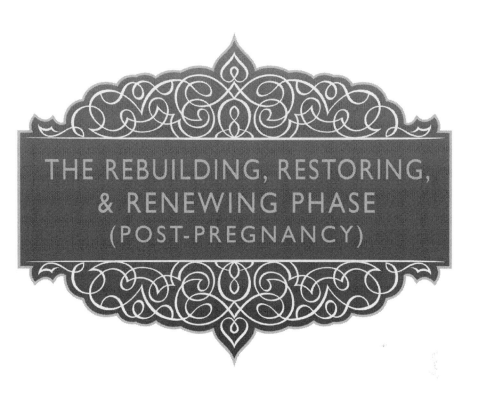

THE REBUILDING, RESTORING, & RENEWING PHASE
(POST-PREGNANCY)

My mother raised me, and then freed me. - Maya Angelou

Doulas, midwives, and wise women from various ethnic cultures in the West refer to the period after birth (and the subsequent six weeks) as the fourth trimester, puerperium and post-natal. *The Rebuilding, Restoring, and Renewing Phase*, as I call it, is as important as any other part of the birthing process. A mother's health is depleted during pregnancy and labor but also after the birth of the baby. She is constantly spending her life force energy; therefore, it's crucial that she replenishes and cares for her health after birth.

Rebuild Your Health

With your digestive power now weakened, you'll have to meet greater nutritional requirements to regain your strength post-birth and breastfeed your newborn baby. An investment in your postpartum recovery, immediately after birth, is a worthy investment for your long-term health.

Many elders have told me that women who neglect their health in their childbearing years—especially after the birth of a baby — are sure to feel discomfort during menopause and may invite chronic disease issues in the body. For example, you may want to indulge on a food item you're craving or enjoy a celebratory feast that may not necessarily be good for you or the baby right after birth. Avoid the temptation to squander this time by rushing back to your pre-pregnancy lifestyle and habits.

Since the baby's intestinal lining is still developing in the first 42 days after birth and your body still needs to heal properly, it is absolutely critical that you follow a sattvic (sentient state of living) diet with Ayurvedic food. Doing this will make breastfeeding and digestion easier for both you and your baby, which will really help your newborn be less fussy.

The sattvic diet is a liquid diet. It is light, carminative, and nutritious — contrary to the sweet, oily, and heavy diet of pregnancy. You can gradually step up from the liquid diet to semi-solid and solid foods by the tenth day after childbirth. By day 30, you can slowly return to your routine diet.

In India, the post-pregnancy period is given much emphasis to allow a mother to recuperate from childbirth and bond with the newborn baby. During this 42-day confinement period, the new mom is also mothered. Her own mother and female relatives care for her while she, in turn, cares for her child. Her primary job is to rest, rejuvenate and replenish. Typically, a new mom would return to her mother's house for the pregnancy, birth, and the postpartum period but if she is unable to do so, then the mother will typically move in with the new mom during this time.

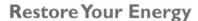

Restore Your Energy

The post-pregnancy phase may be challenging for the modern-day woman since it basically requires that you replace your regular diet with simple foods and update your usual routine to entail little activity for 42 days. It may seem like a big sacrifice to have to follow yet another regimen after already having been restricted for nine to ten months throughout pregnancy—especially when you just want to get back to normalcy.

The good news, we can modify the Ayurvedic postpartum diet by incorporating modern-day techniques with ancient Ayurvedic rituals. Before getting into the how-to's, let's first explore the logic behind the beautiful, ancient cultural traditions that exist to help moms nourish and strengthen their bodies after giving birth.

As Simran Adeniji (Childbirth Educator) says, "In my experience, women who follow this practice — including receiving the help from others — have lower rates of postpartum depression."

What I have learned about ancient traditions, in general, is that these rituals are layered with rich meaning, connection and love. When performed on a new mother, the ceremonies are a celebration of coming together to bolster up and lift a fellow woman in the new endeavor of motherhood. It is very different than the modern-day ritual of checking into a hospital to give birth, then checking out two days later and returning home to be all alone with a newborn baby for the next eight to twelve weeks.

I've spoken to numerous women who've shared with me their regret for not taking care of themselves during this pivotal phase and for not allowing the natural process of motherhood to occur. If you deny yourself the time to restore your energy by rushing to lose weight or return too quickly to your previous lifestyle, the damages can be long-lasting.

Keep your body warm. Only drink warm liquids and foods. Pre-plan frozen meals or get prepared meals delivered to you in bed so that you can get the rest and relaxation you need. Ground yourself. Root yourself back to earth. All of these things can help restore your energy.

Renew Your Life

The desire, in our current culture, to look like a supermodel and be a supermom is unrealistic and self-sabotaging. This is not a judgment about women who choose those goals. However, if an activity does little to support your goals or align with your lifestyle at this time, you must examine the long-term effects of your decisions and reconsider them, if need be.

What if we, new and existing moms, embraced our ancient traditions and found a way to marry them with our modern-day lifestyles? Pregnancy, birth, and beyond could be a time for sisterhood — where we could lean on one another, celebrate, share and ask for help — instead of being so hard on us.

What if we made choices on our terms? Deliberate choices that would allow you to create the space you need to be a more conscious mom and well-rounded woman. This type of outlook and worldview can be a very powerful paradigm shift.

You can control what happens in *your* world simply through the conscious choices you make every day. You can control how you raise your children, how quickly you lose the baby weight, how organic or non-toxic your home is, and how you run your world as the Mother Earth incarnate that you were born to be. Every day, you can be anything you want to be. And if today was less than stellar, you can start over tomorrow. That's the beauty of motherhood.

In "The 42-Day Guide to Caring for Mom after Birth," which is included in the Appendix at the end of the book, you'll learn ways to introduce light as well as simple and non-gas-producing foods into your life that can help you to develop a healthier and happy baby.

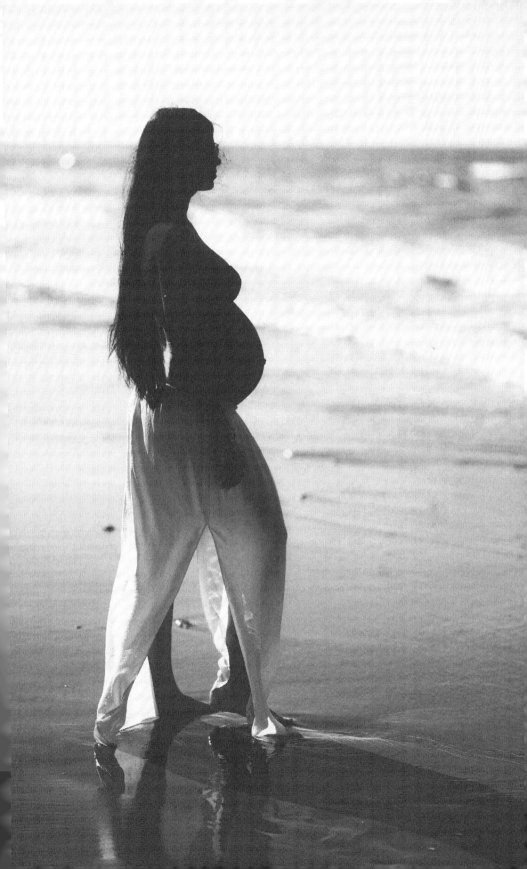

CONCLUSION:

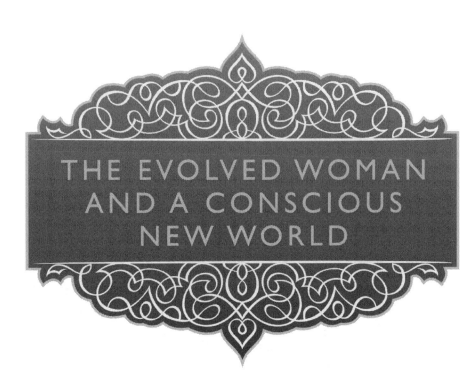

THE EVOLVED WOMAN
AND A CONSCIOUS
NEW WORLD

I'm not afraid of storms, for I'm learning to sail my ship.

- Louisa May Alcott

As you've read up to this point, it's no surprise pregnancy may be the most significant experience you will have as a woman. You'll expand your body, mind, and spirit during this period. You are given the opportunity to explore the abundance of spiritual knowledge and healing practices all around you.

You're creating a spiritual and mental space every day for self-care and you're now prioritizing the time and space for more peace, calm, and joy to enter into your life.

You're taking the time to be quiet and still. You're enjoying meditative practices that help you get deeply relaxed, centered and balanced each day.

You've stopped listening to the fear-based hype and you're turning inward for the truth.

You now appreciate what pregnancy and childbirth symbolize because it's a time to be naturally creative, open-minded, and explorative. Rather than viewing your physical restrictions as a detriment, you're finding the opportunity to open yourself up to activities and mindsets you wouldn't normally practice.

In this new conscious world you've created, your baby is healthy and happy. He or she is born without higher-than-safe levels of BPA in the umbilical cord. The risk of childhood cancer is low. Chances of autism, ADD, ADHD, and learning disabilities have decreased. Your baby is born disease-free and will be raised in a balanced and loving home.

In the West, we have been driven by a strict and fear-based society — fear of liability, fear of experimenting with ancient practices, fear of lacking scientific proof. Conformity and compliance are the consequences.

In Eastern or ancient cultures, many practices and traditions seem non-sensible and superfluous to some. They are archaic in these modern times — today, we seek what actually makes sense and is practical and useful for our life's framework.

In a conscious new world, we combine the best of both worlds. Many belief systems surround us and every one of them would agree that we are striving for a similar new world—one that is more collectively conscious. We've got healers, mediums, therapists, shamans, gurus, chakra readers, Akashic readers, and teachers occupying a whole different space, using tools we don't quite understand.

From the East to the West, we have so much opportunity to learn and grow from each other. We no longer feel powerless about the factors influencing our world: politics, climate change, crime, the community. We acknowledge we may never resolve these problems. However, we know we hold significant power over our state of happiness and ability to improve our quality of living. We can start small and still make ripples in the world.

In this new conscious world, there is another way of doing things. Remember, you are a blank canvas. Take your paintbrush and build that masterpiece. Slow down. Take a deep breath. Deliberately brush each stroke carefully and thoughtfully. Be the Michelangelo of your pregnancy and, in the end, you'll have an illuminating painting—the evolved new you and your Zen Baby.

Acknowledgements

I am so grateful for the incredible man I married and our two beautiful children. Every day, I revel at the bundles of joy we have both created. Our kids are happy, pure, blissful little beings who bring us immense happiness each day. My husband and children truly are the light of my life. Because of them, I have learned more about the universe and myself than I ever imagined possible.

My sister, Neha, my pillar of strength. Aside from being the best sister, she is my best friend. She and I are co-conspirators on many entrepreneurial ventures and together we are making a positive difference in the world. Neha has been an integral part of each of my children's pregnancies and births. She is the best aunt on the planet and my children adore her. She is the kindest and most caring sister in the whole world. I love her dearly for always going out of her way to take care of me when I need her most.

My parents who worked tirelessly to provide a great life for my sister and me. They showed me unconditional love and support throughout my entire life. They encouraged me to pursue my passions—even if it didn't look like a 9-to-5 job—because they wanted me to do what mattered to me. My dad was adventurous when it came to experimenting with new vitamins, organic foods, and green juices. He made a tremendous impact on how I viewed healthy living (this occurred well before the movement towards green living became a trend). After I had finished college, my dad passed away. Family and friends, to this day, reminisce with me about the days he would show up with a different concoction or natural remedy to fix an ailment. My dad instilled this curiosity in me to serve others as a catalyst for conscious living. Much of the foundational knowledge I bring to this book was inspired by his influence.

Kavita, my best friend and sister-in-law. These last five years, Kavita and I have been there for each other. Child after child and pregnancy after pregnancy, we've experimented together figuring out how to raise beautiful and healthy babies in this complex and chaotic world. She is my confidant in life and, through her, I've learned so much about true friendship.

I also want to acknowledge the amazing holistic practitioners out there making a tremendous difference in this world. Some of them are highlighted in this book. For the healers I have not named, I likewise love and appreciate you. Right now, in these modern times, we are blessed to have many modalities we can explore that will work for us and our bodies: acupuncture, chiropractic, Chinese or Western herbal medicine or homeopathy, and other natural healing practices. Thank you for inspiring me.

About the Author

Shivani Gupta was born and raised in Houston, Texas by a loving traditional Indian family. At an early age, she was empowered to make healthy nutritional choices. Her father was the epitome of healthy living. He taught her about organic foods, natural supplements, and how to fortify the body for best health.

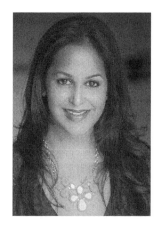

After decades as an ambitious scholar and now an authority on organic living, Shivani is helping women fuel their mind, body, and soul for a conscious pregnancy and Zen Baby. She is an adoring wife, the proud mother of two healthy children, a relentless serial entrepreneur, and scholar of Ayurvedic medicine.

Shivani holds a Master's Degree in Ayurvedic Studies and completes a Ph.D. in Ayurvedic Studies in 2017. Before pursuing Ayurvedic medicine, Shivani studied business at Babson College in Boston, which is ranked #1 for entrepreneurship.

Coming from a long line of entrepreneurs, Shivani specialized in global entrepreneurship, social entrepreneurship, and marketing. In college, she dreamed of opening a health spa that would optimize people's health through exercise, yoga, alternative healing practices, and an on-site organic café. After college, Shivani worked for Canyon Ranch in the Berkshires where she trained with the industry's best leaders on how to run an award-winning health resort and luxury spa while helping people make profound changes in their lives.

After Canyon Ranch, Shivani launched *Sama Baby Organics*, an organic cotton children's clothing line. *Sama Baby* sold in Whole Foods stores and hundreds of boutiques across the United States. Through this successful venture, Shivani gained expertise and notoriety in organic textiles, Azo free dyes, organic baby products, and organic pregnancy. Her work with *Sama Baby* is featured in *Psychology Today, USA Today, Vanity Fair, Whole Foods, American Baby Magazine, Entrepreneur Magazine, The Examiner*, and several other major publications.

Her dedication as a catalyst of conscious living and authority in the organic sector led Shivani to launch Greenista.com, an eco-conscious blog that received favorable reviews from top celebrities, actresses, and Olympic champions.

Today, Shivani is focused on impacting millions of women's lives as an Ayurvedic practitioner and healer, with her books, and through her business, Fusionary Formulas—an Ayurvedic nutraceutical company transforming people's health, mobility, flexibility, and pain.

For free access to Shivani's best strategies, tips, and insights on preparing for a conscious pregnancy and making a Zen Baby, visit TheConsciousPregnancy.com.

For more information on achieving a healthy, green, and organic lifestyle; how to use Modern Ayurveda in your daily life; or to schedule a one-on-one coaching session with Shivani to obtain a personalized plan for pregnancy and beyond, visit ShivaniGupta.com.

***

If you've enjoyed *The Conscious Pregnancy:
A Spiritual and Practical Approach to Creating a Zen Baby*,
please share your honest feedback by leaving
a star rating and review on Amazon.

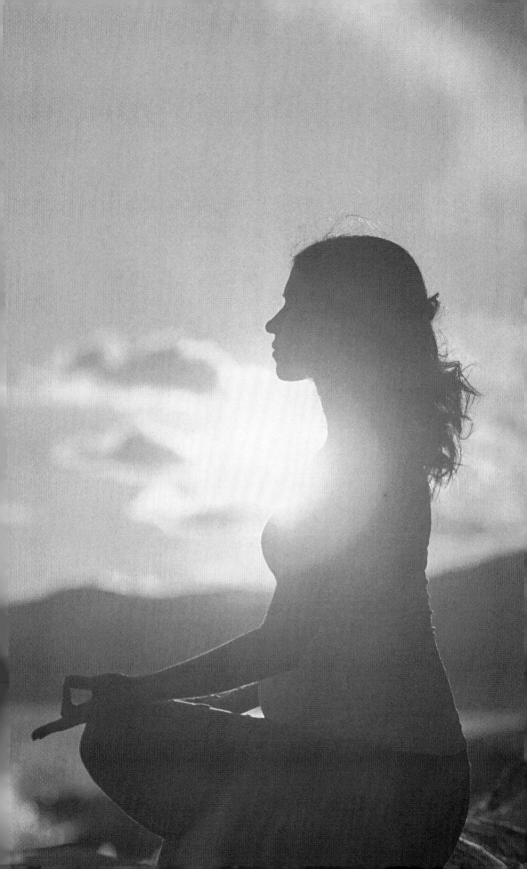

Appendix A:

THE CONSCIOUS PREGNANCY LIFESTYLE CHOICES

Your womb and your baby's growing body are both incredibly sensitive to the world. All around us, we are surrounded by environmental toxins and chemicals. It's in the VOCs lurking in the paint used to remodel your baby's new room. It's in the BPA in those pesky plastic baby bottles. It's even in the pesticides in the conventionally-grown cotton used to make your baby's clothes and toys. Don't become overwhelmed by this information. It's not meant to scare you.

Keep calm, take a deep breath, and feel rest assured you can tackle this. There will be no reason to fear what is completely in your control. You can reduce your exposure to toxins. You have the power to ensure your baby is experiencing minimal exposure as a result of being proactive. You can start cleaning your space, both inside and out, with these ten conscious lifestyle changes.

Stop Using the Microwave

Eliminate your microwave use for anything related to your children and preferably for yourself, especially when you are pregnant. Use your stove or range oven instead.

Clean out Your Beauty Cabinet

Take a look at your beauty cabinet and see what it is in your shampoo, conditioner, body wash, face wash, hand soap, body oil, body lotion, your make-up—everything you put on your body (even your toothpaste or even lip balm, which you ingest).

There are so many layers to the skincare and self-care hygiene routines we have in the morning or evening. As such, there are also many ways to improve these routines by replacing toxic products with less toxic ones.

Learn how to decipher labels so you can avoid artificial fragrances at all costs. Throw out skin care or cosmetic products that contain high levels of toxic ingredients. At the least, switch out the ones that are a priority for you. Do this for hair color and hair care products, make-up, skin care, and dental care. Nix the toxic nail polish. Reconsider conventional sunscreens, bronzers, and moisturizers.

Whole Foods' Whole Body section is a great place to start looking for less toxic solutions. You can use the *Think Dirty* app by founder Liz Tse or the *Skin Deep* app by the *Environmental Working Group*. This app is an excellent resource to quickly research toxicity levels of each product.

To save you time, you can access a list of suggestions and other research we've conducted for you at the book resources page at TheConsciousPregnancy.com.

Switch Out Your Cleaning Products

Many cleaning products are, shockingly, not cleaning your home. These chemicals are actually actively poisoning your home. Switch to a natural solution that will leave less of a toxic burden on your family and will clean up the indoor air quality of your home. Again, use the *Think Dirty* app or *Skin Deep* app to scan for toxicity levels. You can make your own solutions, or visit natural and organic stores for cleaner alternatives.

Eat Fresh Whole Foods

Avoid packaged foods. Food made in a factory uses processes that are more likely to put chemicals in your food. Reduce your consumption of foods that come out of a can, a box, or a plastic bag.

Eat a diet rich in whole foods. You'll feel better when you eat fresh foods. If you must eat packaged foods for convenience, seek out alternatives that are organic or in BPA-free containers. The herbs recommended in an Ayurvedic diet include Ashwagandha (Indian Ginseng), Shatavari (wild asparagus), Gokshur, and Amla (Indian gooseberry).

Some great recipes that include anti-inflammatory Ayurvedic Indian herbs are listed on the book resource page at TheConsciousPregnancy.com.

Choose Toys and Home Goods Made of Natural Materials

Avoid choosing goods for your home that are made of synthetic materials. Choose blankets, textiles, towels and sheets that are made of natural substances. Choose mattresses that aren't doused in flame-retardant chemicals. Choose furniture that is made from sustainable materials. Low VOC or no VOC paint prevents volatile organic compounds from being released into the air. Choose wisely for your décor, flooring, and everything in your home that will come into contact with you and your baby.

Hydrate the Good Way

Avoid soda altogether, especially ones like Mountain Dew. Avoid Red Bull. Drinking sugary drinks that are touting themselves as water is bad for you. Avoid any drinks that are manufactured in a factory.

Choose healthier options. Drink green tea. Drink iced tea. Drink water with fruit in it. Make your own twist of fun, fresh water by adding fruit or lemon. My favorite: lemon and fresh mint.

Explore Alternative Medicine

Stop putting your health care in someone else's hands if you do not agree with their views. If you are not getting the answers you need from your primary care physician or specialist, explore other health and healing alternatives. If you are currently consulting with an alternative healing practitioner and you're not comfortable with the care you're receiving, keep looking.

There is a multitude of alternative medicine and complementary health practitioners in the world with vast amounts of knowledge. You can go to a chiropractor, acupuncturist, homeopath, naturopath, functional medicine doctor, healer, and Ayurvedic doctor. You may have already noticed more hybrid options: a licensed Western medicine doctor also practicing alternative medicine.

Consider all your options and seek out the answers that resonate with you and the solutions you're seeking.

Make Time for Self-Care

Stop letting the mind run its course and abandoning your control over it. Even if you only have five minutes a day, make sure you are making the time to care of yourself. Take small measures to care for your skin, your body, your mind, and your space. Whether it's an abhyanga massage, yoga class, going to the gym, or watching a movie, do what makes you feel good. Find time to listen to music, meditate, go for a peaceful walk, or shut down technology and be alone with your thoughts.

Move Your Body

Get off your butt and stop *trying* to move. Move! Exercise, walk, take a fitness class, do something that revives your energy. Do you like performing? Dance. Sing. Express yourself through art. I assure you, whatever it takes to get you moving your body and exploring the world is nourishing much more than your physical well-being.

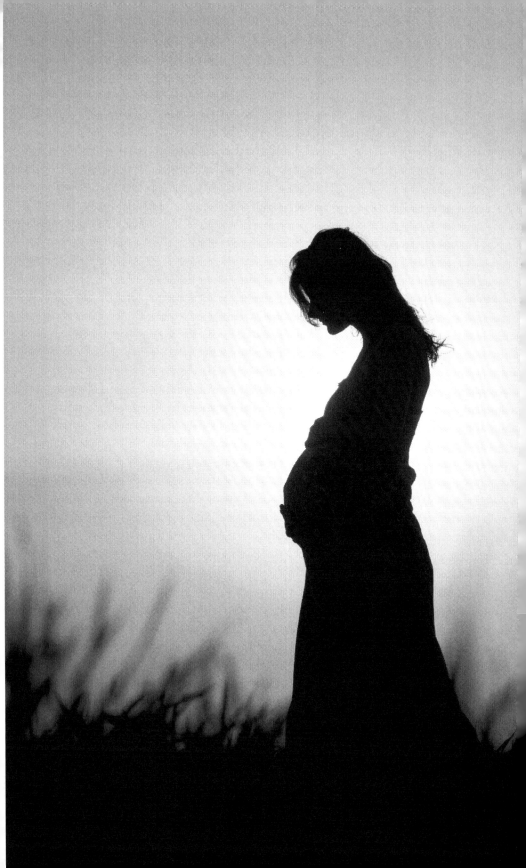

THE CONSCIOUS PREGNANCY DIET GUIDELINES

I'll preface this chapter by saying that *The Conscious Pregnancy Diet Guidelines* is not a fad diet or scheme to help you get quick results. Is it possible to realize immediate results if you follow this plan? Absolutely. However, I urge you to measure your success based on the quality of your long-term health and to focus less on reaping rapid overnight results. The secret to happiness and healthiness is to realize that life is a marathon, not a sprint.

The purpose of *The Conscious Pregnancy Diet Guidelines* is to help you rejuvenate, nourish, and strengthen your body. You can adapt this regimen to accommodate modern-day cooking techniques. And it is important to note that the logic behind many of the ancient cultural health traditions are a big reason why I am keeping many of these guidelines intact.

Make Conscious Nutritional Choices

Science and media are omnipresent, but recently they have been causing more confusion among consumers than ever before. It's no wonder that healthy dieting and nutrition can be hard to grasp. Take a few steps back from all the diet fads and consider a more traditional and global approach to nutrition.

Several cultures have created natural and healthy diets through traditional, whole and nourishing foods. For example, we've got Ayurvedic wisdom (which I've shared in this book) and the classic Mediterranean diet, to name a few. In today's Western culture, we have shunned pure, good sources of sustenance such as healthy fats and dairy. We have deprived ourselves of whole grains in exchange for low-fat, low-carb, and ultimately low-health diets. We've gotten fooled into buying chemically-laden, highly-processed, and hormone-filled foods for the sake of convenience.

Recognizing that the unborn baby is impacted by what we eat, we have got to be more cognizant of the nutritional choices we make before conception, during pregnancy, and while breastfeeding.

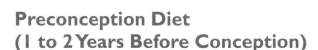
Preconception Diet
(1 to 2 Years Before Conception)

In the simplest terms, a preconception diet is primarily made up of whole foods filled with various plant-based meals.

Creating the ultimate food rules for an ideal preconception diet would look something like this:

IDEAL DIET RULES FOR PRECONCEPTION

Rule #1. Eat plant-based foods, especially greens.

Rule #2. Eat animals treated humanely. These animals have been fed on natural diets and have not been exposed to harmful antibiotics, hormones or preservatives.

Rule #3. Eat the rainbow: Choose a variety of vegetables and fruits with all different colors.

Rule #4. Avoid white bread and processed grains. Stick to whole grains, preferably ones that are sprouted and not hybridized. Choose varieties like einkorn and make sure they are organic. An excellent source of whole grain wheat includes spelt and barley.

Rule #5. Shop along the edges of the grocery store. Stay away from the middle aisles. Avoid the temptation to buy highly-processed foods. These items are loaded with preservatives and added chemicals. Doing so will be the healthier choice and will also help you save a lot of money in the long run.

Rule #6. Buy organic whenever possible. If you're on a budget and can't afford to buy everything organic, do not fret. Check out the EWG's Dirty Thirty and Clean Fifteen for suggestions on how to distinguish between the fruits and vegetables that are sprayed with high doses of pesticides versus ones that are not.

Rule #7. Opt for snacks with unprocessed plant foods. Some great suggestions are carrots with hummus or baba ganoush, unsweetened grass-fed Greek yogurt with seasonal fruits (especially berries), and low-sugar organic granola like Simply Elizabeth.

Rule #8. Limit your sugar intake as much as possible. Sugar exacerbates inflammation in the body and plays a significant role in your microbiome and your newborn baby.

Rule #9. Take a probiotic and eat foods that create healthy gut flora – according to Ayurveda, the gut and the fire inside called agni is the key to good health.

Stop cutting out food groups by going on low-fat or low-carb diets. Instead, focus on quality. Where your food comes from matters because its source impacts your health and well-being. Shoot for higher quality food if you want high-quality health.

How do we measure the quality of food? The quality of food is defined by how it was grown. Was it produced using sustainable or organic practices? Is it non-GMO? Pesticide-free? Hormone and antibiotic-free? Limit your intake of foods that are not nutritious powerhouses (sweets and salty snacks). Maintain a balanced glycemic load to avoid spiking your blood sugar. Research confirms that these approaches to modify your lifestyle will improve your health and decrease your risk of getting most non-communicable diseases—it also improves the health outcomes for your baby.

Ayurveda teaches us to buy the freshest food possible, to never eat leftovers (or eat them sparingly), to use organic foods in our diet, not to use the microwave, and much more.

Conception and Pregnancy Diet (All Trimesters)

During all phases of pregnancy, there is increased demand for food, energy, blood, nourishment, and nutritional supplements like proteins, vitamin, and fats. A few select additions and changes in dietary patterns can benefit the pregnant woman and baby exceptionally.

When we neglect or deprive our physical and mental health, we also abandon our responsibility to contribute to our growing baby's health. An unbalanced diet can lead to miscarriage, premature delivery, or even an underweight baby. Balance your diet with good nutritional value during pregnancy.

Supplementation. As soon as you get pregnant, it's important that you refrain from any new supplementation. In the United States, we have conservative doctors. These physicians must adhere to strict guidelines and work within the liability of their malpractice insurance or the guidelines of their academies. *The American Academy of Obstetrics* and *The American Academy of Pediatrics* both have their own guidebooks, as does The American Academy of pretty much any large medical group.

As a first-time mom, you are new to the whole experience so you might do as you are instructed without understanding all of the other options and alternatives you have. Pregnant women receive a bag full of pharmaceutical samples from their obstetrician. These prescription-grade samples of fish oil, or Omega 3, Omega 6, and prenatal vitamins are not required for a healthy pregnancy; however, we've been firmly advised to take them.

It is a good idea to stop taking supplements in which you are not familiar. Fish oil and pre-natal vitamins are typically safe choices. Many homeopathic, Ayurvedic, and Chinese herbal medicine supplements are safe. Have your practitioner conduct a blood test to identify where your vitamin and mineral levels are deficient or in excess so you can get back to ideal levels before getting pregnant. The onus is on you to talk to alternative practitioners or to do your own research to determine what is safe for you.

Once you become pregnant, your choices are limited and you will have to roll with things as they are. By planning ahead, you have the opportunity to create what you want. You will have greater control over the quality of your pregnancy, childbirth, and future. Analyze where you are right now and what you can do to create a safe haven for your unborn baby.

Postpartum Diet

In India, the postpartum period is a vital time in a woman's life. The new mom must recuperate from childbirth and bond with the newborn baby. During the confinement period, 42 days after childbirth, the baby's digestive lining is still being formed. What goes into mommy's stomach goes right into the baby's breastmilk.

What you eat directly impacts the baby's health, stomach, digestion, mood, and much more. Since your digestive power will be weakened after childbirth, a sattvic diet is recommended. The sattvic diet is a light, carminative, and nutritious liquid diet—contrary to the sweet, oily, and heavy diet of pregnancy. You can gradually step up from the liquid diet to semi-solid and solid foods by the tenth day after childbirth. Once you get to day 30, you can gradually return to your normal diet.

You can find the full resource guide for the post-partum diet guidelines in "Appendix C: The 42-Day 'Taking Care of Mom after Birth' Guide."

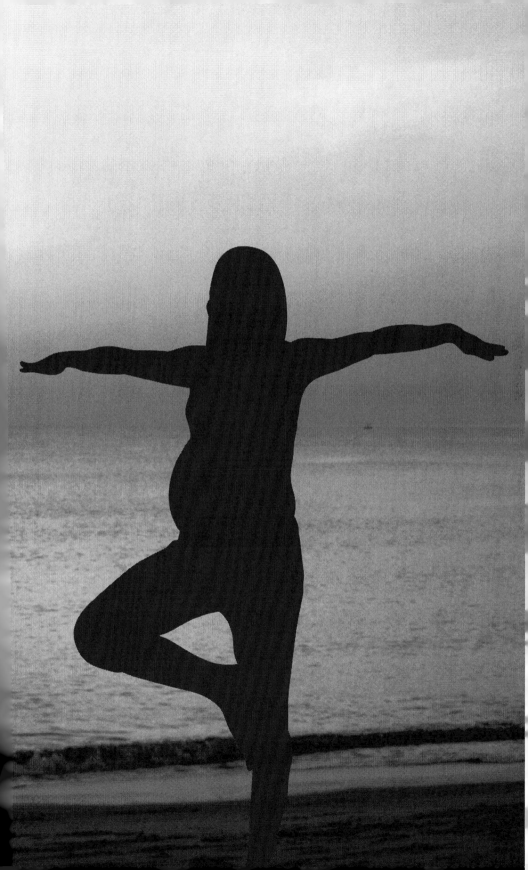

Appendix C:

THE 42-DAY "TAKING CARE OF MOM AFTER BIRTH" GUIDE

The baby's intestinal lining develops in the first 42 days after birth. During this postpartum period, it is important to consume a sattvic diet (an Ayurvedic diet that consists of light, soothing, easily-digestible food) to help mom's body heal. It's best to have all your resources prepared — food and spices in the cabinet ready to go—so there's no extra stress or running around during the next 42 days.

High Vata During Postpartum

The postpartum period is considered high Vata in Ayurveda, which means it's especially important for the new mom to take special care during this time to balance Vata.

What is Vata? One of the central teachings of Ayurveda, the body is made up of different combinations of the primal elements, which are earth, water, fire, air, and ether. These are the life energies behind all of our bodily functions. There are three doshas (*Dosha* is a Sanskrit word meaning "fault" or "defect") in the Ayurvedic principles: Vata, Pitta, and Kapha. According to Ayurveda, each of us (since we were conceived) possesses a unique makeup of Vata (space, air), Pitta (fire, water), and Kapha (earth, water) that creates an individual blueprint for our ideal state of balance. People with a predominance of Vata dosha have quick, creative minds—but they also often forget things just as quickly. They also walk and talk fast but are easily fatigued as they are not very good at holding their energy.

This can be a recipe for disaster if Vata is not balanced during the postpartum period.

During this period of confinement, you can enjoy the following traditional recipes in small portions. Bear in mind, moderation is the key. Many of these recipes are made with a lot of ghee and sugar because these ingredients are believed to provide vital nutrients and aid lactation. For greater balance, mix in healthy vegetarian soups and easy-to-digest meals and proteins.

DAILY MUST-DOS

- Rest, shower, and sleep. That's it. No other activities. No parties or outings.
- Keep the body warm. Wear a hoodie and socks as well as a shawl on your head.
- Have your meals served to you (in a tray) in bed. This allows you to get rest.
- If you are constipated, MiraLAX® is safe to use.

Prepare in Advance

- **Homemade Ghee (clarified butter):** Prepare in advance or order organic ghee online.
- **Special Ghee:** Soak ajwain (also called bishop's weed) in ghee for three weeks. Use this mixture on your tortillas or foods for the 42-day period.
- **Special Water:** Put one spoon of ajwain in one glass of water and boil it a lot. Then, cover and let cool. Water with ajwain spice: sift it, and then drink it from a thermos all day.
- **Atta ka halwa (special Indian dessert to aid lactation):**
  - There are many types of halwa: panjiri halwa, atta ka halwa (made of flour), and badam halwa (made of almonds).
  - This Indian dessert is delicious, sweet, and easy to eat as a snack or even as dessert with a meal

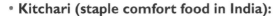

- **Kitchari (staple comfort food in India):**
  - Bulgur wheat (also called Dahlia in North India) is an Indian go-to dish that helps increase milk supply (heavier and excellent for lactation).
  - Green mung beans (for protein).
  - Optional. Add one whole zucchini (lightens the kitchari).
  - Always use specialty Indian spices for their health benefits.

List of Ayurvedic Foods Recommended for the First Few Weeks after Birth

- Legumes: green mung beans, red lentils, yellow mung
- Whole milk dairy products
- Whole grains: well-cooked
- Ghee (clarified butter)
- Nuts/nut butter
- Fruit
- Avocado
- Cooked vegetables (avoid cruciferous vegetables)
- Ginger (in small amounts)
- Cumin, Fenugreek, Fennel, Dill, Basil, Coriander, Mineral Salt
- Milk puddings, tapioca, rice pudding (without eggs)
- Gourds, cooked apples, zucchini, squash, peas, potatoes, carrots, butternut squash, pumpkins, and limited tomatoes are all good
- One glass of fresh paneer (fresh cheese) occasionally
- Nourishing soups with seasonal vegetables (warming to the body)
- After 15 days, you can introduce peas and a small amount of tomatoes
- Black tea and green tea is also fine

LIST OF AYURVEDIC FOODS NOT RECOMMENDED DURING THE FIRST WEEKS AFTER BABY

- Spicy food (can irritate the baby)
- Ginger, garlic, onion, turmeric
- Cucumber, peas, okra, cilantro
- Cruciferous vegetables: cauliflower, Brussel sprouts, broccoli
- Soy
- Yogurt (it's cold). Take acidophilus instead.
- Fermented food
- Rice
- Banana (too heavy)
- Cinnamon
- Lemon and lime (too acidic)

Day One Meal Recommendations (Day of Birth)

- Weak tea
- No cold water after the baby is born. Room temperature only.
- Drink with straw only, or drink slowly.
- Don't drink orange juice, apple juice, or any juices for the first month.
- Drink as much water as you can (eight 8-ounce glasses per day is a good starting point).
- Dahlia, kitchari, or fresh soup (brought from home) at the hospital.

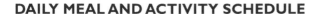

DAILY MEAL AND ACTIVITY SCHEDULE

- **Pre-breakfast:** Special water with ajwain spice in it, multigrain toast, hot milk (sheep, goat, or almond).
- **Morning rest**
- **Breakfast (Option A):** Toast. Halwa (sweet dessert pudding from North India).
- **Breakfast (Option B):** Halwa with chai or warm almond milk. One piece of toast and butter.
- **Lunch:** Kitchari or cooked vegetable with Indian tortilla (Sattvic Foods).
- **Dinner:** Kitchari or cooked vegetable with Indian tortilla (Sattvic Foods).

You can find additional resources online at TheConsciousPregnancy.com.

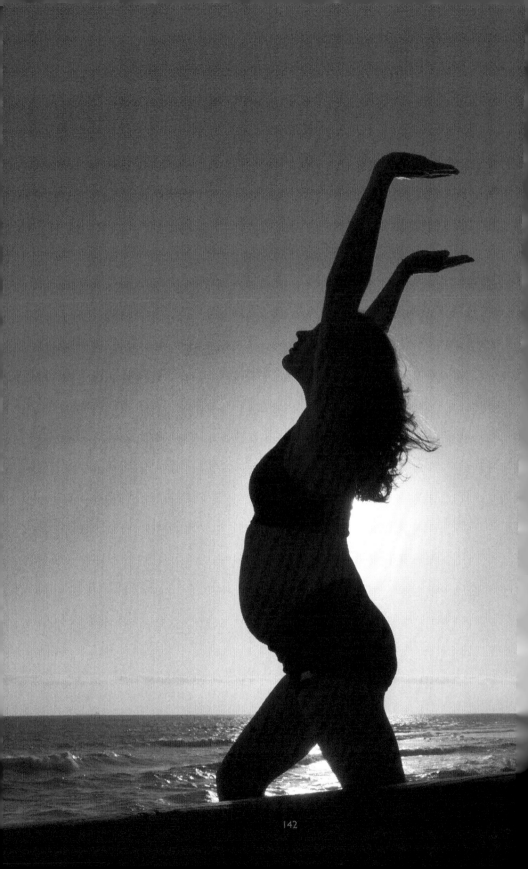

Appendix D:

TERMS, DEFINITIONS, AND RESOURCES FROM THE EXPERTS

There are many terms I've used in the book that may not be clear to the first-time mom. This section elaborates on those frequently used terms and their meanings, as well as providing other resources from experts I know and trust.

FROM LORIE MCCOY ON BIRTHING CENTER SERVICES

WHAT IS A MIDWIFE?

A midwife is someone who:

* Monitors the physical, psychological, and social well-being of the mother throughout the childbearing cycle
* Provides the mother with individualized education, counseling, a nd prenatal care, continuous hands-on assistance during labor and delivery, and postpartum support
* Minimizes technological interventions

- Identifies women who require obstetrical attention and refers them accordingly
- The application of this woman-centered model of care has been proven to reduce the incidence of birth injury, trauma, and cesarean section.

What is a doula?

A doula understands the needs of and supports the new parents at childbirth. Once labor begins, your doula joins you at home and accompanies you to your chosen birthing place, unless you are planning a home birth. She stays with you for the length of your labor and stays one to two hours after the baby is born until you are all settled and breastfeeding has been established.

What is a postpartum doula?

The doula tends to the baby's needs as a baby nurse does, but also is there to reassure and encourage both parents by teaching and mentoring them on how to care for the newborn. The doula assists the parents by teaching them to trust their own instincts in trying to meet their baby's needs. The doula can help tremendously with any first-time parents, especially those without family in the area. Postpartum doulas can also be helpful to parents of multiples, mothers recovering from cesarean births, women experiencing postpartum depression and anxiety, parents of babies with colic or reflux, and babies with special needs.

What is a home birth?

The midwifery model of care is designed to provide one-on-one care to an extent not possible in modern obstetrics. The midwifery model is a minimum standard that strives to provide the most personalized and evidence-based care available for all levels of service.

What is a water birth?

Water birth, which occurs in water, has been both supported and criticized by parent, child, and birthing organizations. Though evidence suggests that water immersion can result in fewer epidurals and adverse effects, there is insufficient information regarding the effects of giving birth in water. Many proponents of water birthing believe it to be a more relaxing and less painful experience that promotes a midwife-led model of care.

What is a birthing center?

A birthing center offers families a safe and effective option for the birth of their child. Parents are carefully screened to ensure that the birthing center services are suited to meet their needs. Women are encouraged to birth naturally with minimal interventions. Postpartum mothers have the option to stay with a certified postpartum doula typically for 24 hours to assist them with breastfeeding.

What is HypnoBirthing®?

According to the HypnoBirthing Institute, HypnoBirthing® The Mongan Method allows women to use their natural instincts to bring about a safer, easier, and comfortable birthing using self-hypnosis techniques. It is presented in a series of five, two-and-a-half hour classes.

What is the Bradley Method®?

What is the difference between The Bradley Method® and other types of childbirth classes? The Bradley Method® of Husband-Coached Natural Childbirth attracts families who are willing to take the responsibility needed for preparation and birth.

Certainly, one of the biggest positives of natural childbirth is the fact that the baby will not be prone to the possible side effects of drugs given during labor and birth. The Bradley Method® classes teach families how to have natural births. The techniques are simple and effective. They are based on information about how the human body works during labor. Couples are taught how they can work with their bodies to reduce pain and make their labors more efficient. Of over one million couples trained in The Bradley Method® nationwide, over 86 percent have had spontaneous, unmedicated vaginal births.

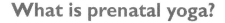

What is prenatal yoga?

Prenatal yoga allows you to adapt gracefully to each phase of this momentous time in your life. The yoga techniques enable you to nurture and open your body throughout every stage of pregnancy. Explore breathing techniques, asanas (postures), and mantras as you prepare mentally, physically and spiritually for the conscious awareness of birth and motherhood.

What is a fertility massage?

The body is ready to conceive when it is free of stress, unwanted hormones, and congestion in the pelvic region. Fertility massage works on all three issues with the combination of acupressure, abdominal massage, energy work, and reflexology.

Stress is prevalent among women with fertility issues. It is absolutely important to reduce stress since it increases the amount of hormones in the body that hinder the implantation of the egg.

An abdominal massage increases blood flow to reproductive organs and breaks up any adhesions within the pelvic region, which can increase fertility, improve ovulation and menstrual cycles, support your hormone balance and immune system, and reduce cysts and fibroids.

What is a prenatal massage?

This soothing massage increases circulation, alleviates tired muscles, improves skin elasticity and reduces water retention. At the end of a prenatal massage, warm aromatherapy towels will be applied to your feet for indulgence and relaxation followed by a warm or cool beverage to send you back to the reality that awaits you.

What is an Invitation-to-Baby massage?

Several natural, safe techniques can help stimulate labor—massage and acupressure are two of them. Massage helps facilitate relaxation with long flowing strokes that calm the mind and body, which are essential for a woman to give birth. Acupressure points are also incorporated, which stimulate the contraction of the uterus. Spleen 6, Kidney 3, Liver 3, and Large Intestine 6 are all areas of focus. An induction massage is only for women who are very close to or past their due dates.

What is a postnatal massage?

A postnatal massage assists the body in returning to the pre-pregnant condition. Rejuvenate and relieve the stress of being a new mama, while also supporting the body's postnatal healing process.

What is placenta encapsulation?

Placenta encapsulation has become a mainstream practice in the past few years. It gives mothers who are perhaps a bit squeamish about consuming their placenta (placentophagy) a palatable way to do so. Many women are recognizing the effects of replenishing their postpartum body after labor with all of the iron, protein, vitamins, and minerals in which the placenta is naturally enriched.

There are now links between placenta encapsulation and reduced postpartum depression and "baby blues," as well as an increased potential in positive breast milk production—both due to the amount of the mother's own hormones found in her placenta.

Many women use this service to increase the chances of breastfeeding success and to help create a peaceful and balanced postpartum experience for the whole family—especially for those who are at a greater risk for postpartum depression and anxiety or with a history of infertility or low milk supply.

Resource: LORIE MCCOY, Doula, OrchidNest.com

FROM DR. RICHA GUNDLAPALLI ON ENERGY MEDICINE AND INTEGRATIVE MEDICINE

What do you wish new moms knew before or during pregnancy?

The first thing I always educate or coach parents on before they plan for pregnancy is their readiness factor: how ready and committed are you and your spouse (or the significant person in your life) to bring a child into the world?

I feel that society has a lack of preparing or coaching first-time couples before conception. Not only is it important that physically they are ready but they must also be emotionally, mentally, and spiritually prepared to bring this new soul or new being on this planet.

I encourage couples to read, take classes, take online workshops, and learn about pre-pregnancy preparation, optimum pregnancy and birth, and a healthy postpartum period.

The following are areas in which I've coached my clients:

MIND, BODY, SPIRIT

- Have you detoxified your body and rejuvenated it?
- Do you have enough vitality, strength, and stamina to sustain a pregnancy?

- Is your mental and emotional state positive or stressed? Stress decreases the blood flow to the child, which affects the child's development in utero.

- Detoxifying is important for the mother, but also for the father's sperm quality. Both mother and father must cut out smoking, drinking, and other bad habits before conception.

- Ayurveda has strong rituals for how you prepare for pregnancy (such as rituals for ideal conception according to astrology, and more).

- Mother and father must tailor their detoxification program to consider their cultural sensitivities and the intensity level of their preparedness.

AIR QUALITY

- In addition to detoxifying the body, it's important to also detoxify the home's indoor air quality.

- HEPA filters, wood floors instead of carpet, open windows often, use non-toxic and no-VOC paint on the walls.

WATER

- Chlorinated water kills the good and bad bacteria in the gut. Change your drinking water, your showerhead, and your whole house system if possible.

- Consider filtered or extra clean water for the baby if you give them formula.

FOOD AND PERSONAL CARE ITEMS

- Eat an organic and clean diet.
- Avoid the Dirty Dozen.
- Wash your fruits and veggies well with soap.
- Consider non-toxic soaps, laundry detergents, cleaning supplies, shampoos, conditioners, and hair gels.

During pregnancy what are some factors moms must look out for?

The hormone changes during pregnancy make you a different person. The parents have to totally embrace the loss of identity they will have once the child is here. Some people get depressed postpartum because of this. Embracing the entire process of pregnancy and parenthood is important.

Recognize the difference between good stress and bad stress; adjust your workload at work accordingly. Everything comes down to your stress management and resilience. If you are in a stressed out state while pregnant (from personal stress, relationship stress, or work stress), saying yes when you should be saying no is not good for you or the baby. Stress kills away the good bacteria you have. It also changes your hormone pathways of adrenaline, epinephrine, and cortisol—which causes a lot of inflammation in your body.

High stress = high inflammation = slower wound healing.
Since your healing post-baby is affected by your state of being during
pregnancy, it's imperative to activate the parasympathetic nervous system
(your nurturing and healing nervous system) as much as possible. Take a
nature walk, nurture yourself, indulge yourself, go for a picnic, meditate, use
essential oils, do yoga or any stretching meditation. Doing these things will
produce a healthy, happy child.

Society bombards us with noises, videos, negative stuff on the news,
and work—it is too high stress. Switch your mind and body from stressed
out survival mode to the mode of abundance, safety, and security, which is
very important.

How do you engage your parasympathetic nervous system?
Touch, hold, or caress somebody. Meditate or get a massage. You can also
stimulate the child's nervous system by listening to classical music, learning
a language or new skill, reading, or taking art classes.

What is the role of energy medicine in pregnancy?

If you look into Chinese acupuncture, we have meridians. If you look
into Ayurveda, we have marma points (they call it nadis), which are energy
pathways that nurture your organs in your body—even the baby inside the
womb has these energy pathways.

These pathways, which can even be formed before conception, can sometimes get blocked. When they are blocked, it is like a clot in your blood vessels. The energy does not circulate, similar to when blood circulation stops. It is important to keep these channels clear so that the energy force, the life force, can flow smoothly into the mother and also into the child.

When I consult a pregnant woman or even women who are preparing for pregnancy, I check to see if the mom's template is balanced and clean.

I teach different breathing techniques, meditation and healing techniques to revitalize the mom's health energetically so that the child has a fertile and healthy ecosystem from which to grow. You can be a happy pregnant woman and all of these emotions can activate your parasympathetic nervous system, which is what we want during labor.

With all of the cases I have studied and seen, you do not need as much pain medication if you have a healing coach helping you during the process of labor. My experience as an energy medicine specialist is to do the back end support. I not only work on the parent but also on the family to support the entire unit—it's about getting everyone ready and helping them transition behind the scenes.

What is energy medicine or chakra healing?

As a human being, we have an energy field called the biofield, which is not visible—making it hard to understand. The biofield governs our organ health, emotional health, and mental health. It is like the EKG. We have the electric charge that comes from your heart, which we can measure. There is also an electric charge from your brain, which we can measure. Every cell in your body has its own actual potential and its own charge.

As an energy medicine teacher, what I bring to light is the focus on these energy biofields that we are made up of or that we all have. It is important to care for these energy fields because they govern your entire well-being.

If you can see yourself as an energy field, the chargers have information — they have intelligence. It is like a radio wave. You can tune into any radio wave to listen to the radio. We are like spiritual technology or energy technology. These energy pathways govern your physical body health, your organs, and your endocrine system. They also govern your emotional cleanliness, emotional calmness, or emotional balance to make less reactive decisions. They help you to have more clarity and focus of your mind. They can also help you have the inspiration to move forward in life.

Resource: RICHARITHA GUNDLAPALLI, MD, ABIHM, Board Certified Physician, Integrative Practitioner, Energy Medicine Expert, Certified Life Coach, Social Entrepreneur

FROM MIRANDA CASTRO ON HOMEOPATHY

What is homeopathy?

Homeopathy is an increasingly popular alternative system of healing whose basic philosophy has attracted much skepticism from the conventional medical world because it has been difficult to prove 'scientifically'. However, its success with patients has resulted in continual growth and development over the past two hundred years and homeopathy has seen a significant spike in popularity in the past 20 years.

How does homeopathy treat the patient?

Homeopathic treatment, like all natural therapies, seeks to stimulate the innate healing power of the individual so that all systems can function at their best. As a person moves toward their optimal level of general health, they feel better about themselves. As their symptoms improve, their body's defenses strengthen and become more active.

Minimum dose. As little medicine as possible is employed. After a dose is given the individual's response is carefully observed, and the remedy is repeated or changed as necessary.

Is homeopathy safe in pregnancy?

The safety of homeopathic medicines in pregnancy has been confirmed by 200 years of homeopathic clinical practice with millions of patients all around the world. Although we don't know exactly what the unborn baby of a hurt mother is going through, we do know it will almost certainly affect her child if the mother is in a state of shock. Anything that can help the mother to heal—to feel better in herself must and will be of benefit to the baby.

What is one of your favorite remedies?

I am a self-confessed Arnica fanatic and have been known to wax lyrical about its miraculous properties to anyone who will listen. Arnica works on almost anybody. It is as close to specific as we can get (a specific medicine is one with a high degree of certainty to help with a certain complaint) and we, homeopaths, don't have many of those.

Arnica provides incontrovertible proof that homeopathy works for many people because, as a healing concept, it's fairly fantastic. The idea that anything so small can have an effect is weird because we have to see it to believe it. But once you have seen it work, you will become hooked.

It is somewhat impressive to see that egg on your child's forehead, caused by a nasty fall, quickly reduce and disappear altogether, in front of your very eyes, within minutes ... having only given him or her a single tablet of Arnica (in potency of course). There is no further pain or discoloration. The bruising is healed from the inside. A mini-miracle.

The typical Arnica patient says they are okay when they plainly aren't, and this symptom alone can guide you to a successful Arnica prescription — where there is bruising to soft tissues (muscles) with sore, bruised pains.

When a pregnant woman takes a homeopathic remedy, we can assume that her unborn baby receives something of the same remedy (even if it is a secondary effect). Logically speaking, if a woman is feeling unwell or is hurt, and the remedy stimulates her vital force, her inner healer, then this positive response can only be of benefit to her baby. Arnica alone is a little wonderful remedy during pregnancy. It is used for minor injuries or the discomfort and soreness that comes along with an active baby who kicks, during labor (where it can speed labor and help the muscles to do their work with minimal physical stress and strain), and after the birth by healing strained tissues. Use Bellis perennis for times when Arnica isn't as helpful as expected. Learn your remedies and use them wisely and they will become dear, old friends you cannot imagine ever having lived without!

Resource: MIRANDA CASTRO, FSHom(UK), CCH, RSHom, Best-selling author of Homeopathy for Pregnancy, Birth and Your Baby's First Years

Made in the USA
San Bernardino, CA
25 January 2020